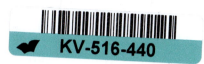

Edited by
ROBERT PEVELER
ELEANOR FELDMAN
TREVOR FRIEDMAN

Liaison Psychiatry

Planning Services for Specialist Settings

RY

GASKELL

© The Royal College of Psychiatrists 2000

Gaskell is an imprint and registered trade mark of the Royal College of Psychiatrists, 17 Belgrave Square, London SW1X 8PG

British Library Cataloguing-in-Publication Data
A catalogue record for this book is available from the British Library.
ISBN 1-901242-47-1

Printed in Great Britain by Bell & Bain Limited, Glasgow.

Contents

iv *Contents*

Contributors

Jennifer Barraclough Formerly Consultant in Psychological Medicine, Sobell House, Churchill Hospital, Oxford OX3 7LJ

Christopher Bass Consultant Liaison Psychiatrist and Honorary Senior Clinical Lecturer, John Radcliffe Hospital, Oxford OX3 9DU

Fiona Blake Consultant Psychiatrist, Addenbrooke's Hospital, Cambridge CB2 2QQ

Jose Catalan Reader in Psychiatry, Imperial College, and Honorary Consultant Liaison Psychiatrist, South Kensington and Chelsea Mental Health Centre, London SW10 9NG

Eleanor Feldman Consultant Liaison Psychiatrist and Honorary Senior Clinical Lecturer, John Radcliffe Hospital, Oxford OX3 9DU

Trevor Friedman Consultant Liaison Psychiatrist, Leicester General Hospital, Leicester LE5 4PW

Julia Gledhill Clinical Research Fellow, Academic Unit of Child and Adolescent Psychiatry, Imperial College School of Medicine (St Mary's), Norfolk Place, London W2 1PG

Elspeth Guthrie Senior Lecturer in Psychiatry and Honorary Consultant Psychiatrist, Manchester Royal Infirmary, Manchester M13 9WL

Andrew Hodgkiss Consultant Liaison Psychiatrist, St Thomas' Hospital, London SE1 7EH

Allan House Professor of Liaison Psychiatry, University of Leeds School of Medicine, Leeds LS2 9LT

Navneet Kapur Lecturer in Psychiatry, University of Manchester, Manchester M13 9WL

Geoffrey Lloyd Consultant Liaison Psychiatrist, Royal Free Hospital, London NW3 2QG

Richard A. Mayou Professor of Psychiatry and Honorary Consultant Psychiatrist, University of Oxford, Department of Psychiatry, Oxford OX3 7JX

Margaret Oates Senior Lecturer and Honorary Consultant Psychiatrist, Queen's Medical Centre, Nottingham NG7 2UH

David Owens   Senior Lecturer in Psychiatry and Honorary Consultant Psychiatrist, University of Leeds School of Medicine, Leeds LS2 9LT

Robert Peveler   Professor of Liaison Psychiatry, University of Southampton, Southampton SO14 OYG

David Protheroe   Specialist Registrar in Psychiatry, General Infirmary at Leeds, Leeds LS1 3EX

Amanda Ramirez   Professor of Liaison Psychiatry, Guy's and St Thomas' Hospital Trust, London SE1 7EH

Michael Sharpe   Senior Lecturer in Psychological Medicine, University of Edinburgh, Honorary Consultant Psychiatrist, Royal Edinburgh Hospital, Edinburgh EH10 5HF

David Storer   Consultant Psychiatrist, General Infirmary at Leeds, Leeds LS1 3EX

Preface

The provision of liaison psychiatry services in the UK, and indeed in much of Europe, is patchy. This suggests that there are difficulties in developing such services. Why should this be? Over the past 20 years, much research has highlighted the possible clinical benefits of liaison services, yet getting this research into practice continues to prove particularly difficult. There seem to be special problems relating to the development of such services within current health care models.

In the UK, the past decade has witnessed the arrival of the purchaser/provider split, an increased emphasis on purchasing led by primary care and separation of specialist hospital services from community and mental health services within different provider organisations ('trusts'). Liaison psychiatry services thus find themselves operating in the 'cracks' between other services, with no obvious line of accountability nor a clear 'market' in which to develop and 'sell' services. There is also confusion about the nature of the product that is being provided, with considerable variation in the way services are organised and focused. In some districts, activity is confined to managing deliberate self-harm, while in others such work is done by community teams and liaison services are focused on attachments within medical or surgical specialities, such as oncology.

The Liaison Psychiatry Section of the Royal College of Psychiatrists works to try to strengthen clinical activity and research in this field. In 1994 the precursor to the current volume was published, entitled *Liaison Psychiatry: Defining Needs and Planning Services*. This outlined the groundwork required for developing core services and establishing local needs. The present volume complements this, with emphasis on more specialist areas of liaison psychiatry practice. We hope that, together, the two books will help practitioners to argue the case for their services more effectively and persuasively. The ultimate goal is to see better-developed services meeting the needs of patients more effectively and efficiently.

1 Developing services in liaison psychiatry: making the case of need

ROBERT PEVELER and ALLAN HOUSE

Consultation–liaison psychiatry concerns the provision of psychiatric services to general hospital patients. There is growing evidence that such services make a major contribution to the quality of patient care. This is summarised in the joint reports of the Royal Colleges of Physicians (Royal College of Physicians & Royal College of Psychiatrists, 1995) and Surgeons (Royal College of Surgeons, 1997) with the Royal College of Psychiatrists, which stress the importance of providing adequate services for the psychological needs of medical and surgical patients. However, at present in the UK National Health Service (NHS), such services are far from uniformly developed, and further action is required.

The NHS reforms in 1991 radically altered the processes of planning and service development. The main changes were the separation of the commissioning function (passed to integrated local health authorities and general practitioner fund-holders) from the provider function (fulfilled by multiple independent hospital and community trusts), the abolition of the regional health authorities, and the move towards a primary-care-led health service. The 'internal market' required that providers of services produce business plans, which became central to the contracting process. Further reform following the 1997 White Paper *The New NHS: Modern, Dependable* is now in progress, but the changes are less radical than those of 1991, and the general principles of an internal market and primary-care-led commissioning look set to stay, with primary care groups leading the commissioning of secondary care services. As a result, anyone wishing to develop a consultation–liaison psychiatry service within the NHS is faced with the need to create a new case of need, yet few clinicians have received any training in this process. As a response to

1

this, the Liaison Psychiatry Section within the Royal College of Psychiatrists held a workshop to improve understanding of the processes involved and generate advice for clinicians faced with this task. This chapter is based upon the output from that workshop.

The aim of this opening chapter is to outline the general principles of developing a case of need for a liaison psychiatry service. Subsequent chapters deal in greater detail with the issues facing different types of specialist liaison psychiatry services. The planning context is outlined below and the business planning process is described. The important ingredients of a case of need are then defined and the process of developing the case is summarised.

Understanding the context

In order to develop a successful case of need for a new service, it is vital to understand the planning context. Before 1991, services developed in an incremental but disjointed fashion according to the availability of resources, progress in the current state of medical knowledge and the balance of power in the local medico-political environment. Planning concentrated upon *inputs*, such as numbers of beds or staff, rather than *outputs*, such as health gain. Now the emphasis has shifted towards the investment of resources for the attainment of defined objectives and outcomes, and provider units are encouraged to develop a corporate strategy to do this. Previously, planning exercises occurred in isolation, with a narrow focus on the service being developed; now attention must be paid to the whole service and any knock-on effects of new developments.

The local context

The planning process involves a complex and confusing network of individuals and organisations, including both the commissioners and providers of health care, and it is essential to assess the local picture before preparing the case of need, identifying local priorities and sources of influence. Increasingly, general practitioners play a major role in the commissioning of secondary care services and are involved in the assessment of provider unit cases of need. The person preparing the document must try to adopt the perspective of the individuals who will be involved in assessing the value of the proposed service. When writing a case of need, clinicians are likely to assume a level of knowledge and understanding greater than that which is actually possessed by the commissioners of services. This is particularly so for consultation–liaison psychiatry, which is a complex model of service provision, usually involving more than one provider unit (mental health and acute medical trusts). A clear description of the clinical problems and possible methods of meeting health needs will be required. 'Consumer' views are also given high priority when reviewing cases of need and should be taken into account.

The national context

The case of need must identify clear aims and objectives for the service that are both achievable and measurable. The outcomes sought must not only be consistent with the broad aims of local commissioning groups and trusts, but should also dovetail with national policies, such as those set out in the 1998 Green Paper *Our Healthier Nation*. There is now great emphasis on the 'appropriateness' of treatment and, while a precise definition of this concept is lacking, the general notion of maximising 'health gain' for a given resource input informs all commissioning decisions. The principal tasks for the person preparing the case of need are therefore to specify clearly what positive outcomes for patients can be expected and to ensure that these can be achieved (and can be shown to have been achieved) at the lowest possible cost.

Ideally, a range of options for service development should be outlined (including the 'do nothing' option), rather than just one preferred method of service delivery. It is vital to explain why the service proposed cannot be provided within existing resources and to highlight the contribution of specialist skills to patient care. For many clinicians, a 'paradigm shift' is needed: we are used to thinking of the development of a *speciality*, but must now think in terms of developing a *service*. The training needs of staff must be fitted into the service model – as opposed to their training experience dictating the shape of the service, as has happened in the past. Explicit justification for each staff member will be needed, including the reasons for developing a service that is medically led.

Current levels of provision

The current state of existing services will also have a bearing on the way in which the planning proceeds. At present, well developed services are mostly found in the larger teaching hospitals, located in urban areas. Such areas may have at best a static level of funding, dictating that any service development can occur only if there is corresponding disinvestment in existing services, maximising health gain for an existing unit of resource. Smaller units in rural areas are more likely to receive some new investment and there may be greater scope for service development here, although any new funding is likely to be closely tied to the strategic aims and objectives of commissioners.

Any case of need has two hurdles to overcome. First, commissioners must be persuaded that the service is worth commissioning. However, as most commissioners cannot afford to purchase everything they wish to, the second hurdle is to persuade them that the service is of sufficiently high priority for it to be included in investment plans. It is therefore important to establish *relative* merit as well as absolute merit.

The planning process

Since the advent of primary care groups, there has been local variability in the way in which the planning process proceeds. Usually commissioners will produce only broad strategies for service development, leaving detailed planning and service specification to providers. Clinical directorates will already have existing business plans, updated annually, which include a specification of the level of service currently provided and an indication of the volume of activity contracted for, together with a contract price. Service developments require the preparation of a new case of need that justifies the need for the new service and defines its costs, benefits and levels of activity.

Many trusts have a template for cases of need; an example is shown in the Appendix. Such a case of need will start life within a clinical directorate, but at this first hurdle difficulties specific to consultation–liaison psychiatry arise, because a number of different clinical directorates will ultimately have to be involved in the process. Services around the country vary, but probably the most common model is that liaison services will be provided by a mental health trust (or directorate) on a service agreement to the acute trust (or directorate). There are instances of services being developed by acute medical provider units; however, it is necessary to ensure that the case of need under development fits with existing provider business plans and is incorporated in the trust's corporate strategy and objectives, as agreed by the trust board. For liaison services this will usually involve more than one trust.

The 1997 White Paper described 'Health Improvement Programmes', which appear to be similar in scope to current 'purchasing intentions' documents, although precise details of the new arrangements were unclear at the time of writing and in any case are likely to vary locally. Different arrangements are likely to be made in Scotland, Wales and Northern Ireland.

Consultation

Consideration must be given to all professional groups involved in, or affected by, the service development: failure to consult with other disciplines is likely to result in failure of the case of need when it arrives at board level. Thought must be given to the skill mix required for the service and an option appraisal of different models of service provision is preferred to an inflexible model. It is best to start with an outline document and to add flesh to the bones as the consultation process proceeds.

Finance

Early consideration must be given to the financial implications of the case of need and it is therefore vital that managerial staff are involved in developing the costings from the beginning. As outlined above, the context of the existing service will have a bearing on this and any scope for cost savings in other areas must be identified. Once again, special problems occur for liaison psychiatry, because savings are most likely to accrue to a different directorate or trust from that providing the service (e.g. shorter length of stay of overdose patients in medical wards).

The evidence that liaison psychiatry services can yield cost savings (House, 1995; Royal College of Physicians & Royal College of Psychiatrists, 1995) should be cited. Without good evidence, the task of persuading commissioners to fund the development of liaison services is difficult, although where published evidence is scant, national or even local consensus can be a potent force, as long as it is not seen as simply a reflection of the vested interests of certain groups. The Cochrane Library (Update Software, Oxford) can provide a useful source of up-to-date reviews of evidence.

Ingredients of the case of need

(1) Product definition

A perceived weakness of liaison psychiatry is that its scope and methods are not sufficiently well defined. An important task for the speciality is to rectify this, and the development of a new case of need provides a useful opportunity to consider exactly what can be achieved using the specialist skills and knowledge of the liaison psychiatrist. Many units are now adopting the term 'psychological medicine', which, although it has many drawbacks, at least avoids the administrative definition of 'liaison' psychiatry (the newer term defining *what* is done, rather than *where* it is done). Although often decried, some form of concise statement about the aims of the service is helpful. It is important to distinguish the service from the acute adult mental health service for the district. So-called mission statements are often too vague, but a useful example might be:

> The overall aim of the psychological medicine service is to ensure that optimum psychosocial care is available to all adult in-patients and out-patients in the general hospital.

The *core* components of such a service will usually include assessment and management both of deliberate self-harm patients and of patients with psychological problems in acute medical and surgical wards as well as the accident and emergency department. Specific liaison services for children and the elderly may be developed in parallel or independently. In addition, a range of other activities may be undertaken, depending on the local environment. It may be useful to categorise these as follows:

(a) services for particular clinical problems – such as unexplained physical symptoms or sexual dysfunction;
(b) services linked to other specialist clinics – such as those provided for pain management or chronic fatigue syndrome;
(c) liaison links with other major units, to provide, for example, psycho-oncology or neuropsychiatry services;
(d) in some liaison services, provision of staff support may also be included, offering, for example, trauma debriefing or a consultation service for work-related mental health problems.

Decisions need to be made about certain services that may form part of liaison psychiatry's remit or that may be provided by others. Examples include general hospital presentations of alcohol and drug dependency (especially involving analgesics), eating disorders and mental illness related to childbirth.

As a first step, it may be helpful to prepare a briefing document on the nature and scope of psychological medicine for local consultation, including something on the frequency and outcome of the common problems dealt with by liaison services. It should be remembered that to stand any chance of being read by its intended audience, the document must be concise and free of jargon. Because of the current emphasis on community services, one helpful way of conceptualising the service may be to portray the general hospital as an additional 'sector' of the community, with special needs that are usually poorly met by existing services. A policy decision needs to be taken about whether a global case of need should be developed for all parts of the service, or whether it would be better to develop specific cases for services to individual units within the general hospital.

Where two trusts are involved (usually a psychiatry or community trust and an acute trust), it is vital to convince managers of both that they have something to gain from the proposed development. The general psychiatry service will be able to manage the general hospital workload more efficiently and may gain in income. The medical trust will gain from improved access to psychiatric services, increased efficiency of bed utilisation, improved quality of medical and psychiatric care, and better management of medico-legal risk.

Psychiatric factors are important in determining the economic outcome of treatment, especially in such areas as cost of care, utilisation of resources and length of hospital stay and quality of life (Saravay *et al*, 1991; Savoca, 1999). Mental health problems that have been shown to influence resource use in hospitals include: cognitive impairment; mood disorder, either anxiety or depression; alcohol misuse; and somatisation. A number of studies from the USA have shown that psychiatric treatment is followed by reduction in in-patient and out-patient resource utilisation. Savings from the reduction in medical service have even been enough to pay for the psychiatric programme, the so-called cost offset effect. Most providers and purchasers will not be familiar with these arguments, which may be best illustrated with case examples, which are often compellingly familiar to clinicians.

In addition to clinical work, a psychological medicine service should play a major role in training medical, nursing and other staff about psychological issues in general hospital patients, again with the emphasis on improving quality. Issues for training will include communication skills, recognition and detection of psychological morbidity, referral protocols to specialist services and techniques for dealing with disturbed behaviour. It should be noted that such educational activity usually results in increased referrals. The service also needs to relate to any other local initiatives for improving aspects of psychosocial care, such as the development of specialist nurses, counsellors and other therapists.

Psychological medicine can also contribute to the trust's research and development profile, either through the conduct of primary research into relevant psychiatric problems, such as somatisation or deliberate self-harm, or through collaboration that adds a psychosocial dimension to research into physical illness.

(2) Choice of outcome measures

A case of need must include a clear statement of its aims and objectives, described in terms of meeting the health needs of defined patient groups. This statement must be supported by clear mechanisms for monitoring the success of the service in attaining its goals and this requires consideration of suitable outcome measures. A wide range of possible indices of performance exist and choice should be informed where possible by local as well as national priorities. The relative importance of each measure will change with both time and place. Possible outcomes include:

(a) avoidance of unnecessary/inappropriate medical admission or investigation;
(b) reduction of readmission (e.g. following deliberate self-harm);
(c) reduced length of stay in hospital (e.g. by contributing to discharge planning);
(d) reduced length of trolley waits in accident and emergency departments;
(e) reduction of complaints related to poor communication;
(f) identification and meeting of unmet mental health needs within the general hospital
(g) improvement in the functional status of patients.

The main emphasis of the case of need is likely to be upon improving quality of care. Further work is needed on the development of appropriate and efficient methods of assessing outcome in this context. The Nuffield Institute for Health at the University of Leeds (which formerly hosted the UK outcomes clearing house) maintains a database of measures and current research in this area, which is available on the World Wide Web and is a good starting point (http://www.leeds.ac.uk/nuffield/infoservices/UKCH/home.html).

It is important to remember that the collection of monitoring data has a cost, which must also be budgeted for in the case of need.

(3) Mention of relevant policies

A very large number of policy documents exist within the NHS, at national, regional, local and trust level, and it is essential to be familiar with these when preparing a case of need so that it may be tailored to prevailing priorities as closely as possible. National documents and initiatives include the planning and priorities guidance from the NHS Executive (although the future of this is now uncertain), *Health of the Nation Mental Health Key Area Handbook* (Department of Health,

1994) and the White Paper *Caring for People: Community Care in the Next Decade and Beyond* (Department of Health, 1989). These are supplemented by the recent publication of *The National Service Framework for Mental Health* (Department of Health, 1999). Trends such as the growth of evidence-based medicine and emphasis on incorporation of recent research findings into clinical practice should be noted, as well as initiatives in areas such as clinical audit, junior doctors' hours, the Calman reforms of medical training and the health of the NHS workforce. The Patients' Charter, and local standards based upon it, should be consulted.

One very important document already mentioned is the joint report of the Royal Colleges of Physicians and Psychiatrists on the shared care of psychological problems in medical patients (Royal College of Physicians & Royal College of Psychiatrists, 1995). The Royal College of Psychiatrists has also published guidance on standards for the management of deliberate self-harm (Royal College of Psychiatrists, 1994).

Regional documents are now less important, but local health authorities may still receive some regional guidance on specific matters such as medical staffing, and outputs from regional research and development programmes may be influential.

Most health authorities have mental health strategies. In addition, at present they publish their commissioning intentions each summer/ early autumn and are likely to continue to do this in some form. These documents are vital in assessing the local picture and give a clear impression of the priorities of local commissioners. Most authorities are concerned about equity, effectiveness and responsiveness of services and about the distinction between health *needs* and *demands*. They will usually ask what health needs are being met by any proposed service, rather than looking for evidence that there is demand for such a service. General practitioners involved in commissioning may, however, have a stronger focus on local demand, as expressed by their own patients. Trusts also focus on demand as a way of assessing business opportunities. Individual fund-holding practices and consortia may produce their own strategy documents and standards.

Aspects of trust policies which may usefully inform the development of the case of need may include risk analysis and risk management policies (e.g. in the management of deliberate self-harm), mechanisms for handling patient complaints (e.g. when a psychiatric problem has been poorly managed in an acute medical ward, or when there has been poor communication) and strategies for meeting the information needs of patients (e.g. giving advice about psychological problems to patients with physical disease).

Writing the case of need

It should now be clear that a case of need must be carefully tailored to the circumstances in which it will be developed and that its development is a complex process involving many people, not just a matter of writing a single document. Personal relationships are likely to be more important than written materials. The document itself will evolve and will spawn a family of related documents, including a definition of the 'product' for wide consultation, an internal trust case-of-need proposal developed with managers and other professional groups, and a final document for submission to the commissioners. Most often the final approach to the commissioners will be in the form of a joint case of need from both mental health and acute provider units. It is important to remember that most trusts have several commissioners and also that a mental health trust may have different commissioners from the acute trust with which it is working.

A successful document will be fully informed by the local context and will conform to any local template. It will usually be helpful to contrast local service provision with the national situation, policies and priorities. The document must be prepared with the target audience clearly in mind, using appropriate, jargon-free language and defining technical terms clearly. An executive summary is an essential feature and often this will be the only part of the document that is actually read! As clinicians are likely to overestimate the knowledge and understanding of managers and commissioners, asking colleagues to review early drafts is vital. It will also be helpful to enlist the help of colleagues in other districts or through networks such as the Liaison Psychiatry Section of the Royal College of Psychiatrists.

The document should include a clear description of the aims and objectives of the service and identify projected improvements in efficiency and health gain. It is then desirable to describe options for attaining the goals and to review the strengths and weaknesses of each, not forgetting the 'do nothing' option. Each option should be considered with regard to benefits, costs and repercussions for other services. It is vital to highlight the costs of *not* developing the service. An internal trust document can include more discussion and debate than a document intended for commissioners. Close attention must be paid to the competencies required of team members in the new service, highlighting necessary knowledge, skills and experience.

Brevity is important – as a rough guide the document should not exceed six pages. Statements not supported by evidence will weaken the document, so full referencing is advisable, possibly in an appendix. Remember though that lay values and patient preferences may carry as much weight as scientific rigour. A concise executive summary and full use of numbered paragraphs and subheadings will assist readability. Innovative methods of getting the message across, such as a video including patient and staff interviews, are worth considering as a means of increasing impact.

As already emphasised, methods of measuring outcome should be detailed and the cost of collecting this information should be included in the overall costing of the service. Capital costs must be detailed separately from revenue.

Identifying the audience and consulting stakeholders

It is vital that the audience for the case of need is identified at an early stage and all potential 'stakeholders' in the process are involved from the beginning. Groups to consider include general psychiatry colleagues (who may oppose development of services in competition with their own), opinion leaders among general medical and surgical colleagues, accident and emergency department staff, specialist nurses within the general hospital, social work departments, service managers, trust board members, representatives of public health and contracting departments within the health authority, and general practitioners.

Clinical audit departments should also be contacted, as helpful supportive data (e.g. patient numbers) may already be available, or readily obtainable. Patient groups should be consulted – for example local branches of MIND. The community health councils still have an important power of veto over changes in service provision and so may undermine developments if not consulted.

Next steps

The preparation of the case-of-need document is the beginning, not the end of the development process. Careful consideration must be given to the way in which the document is disseminated. Besides submission to the commissioners, additional canvassing will be required with local opinion leaders (both clinical and managerial) from both primary and secondary care. However good the document, personal and professional relationships will usually be the principal determinants of success or failure in the service development.

It is important not to be disheartened if the case of need fails on its first attempt – this is a common outcome. Most new cases of need are presented two or three times before being funded and further negotiation is usually required. *Do not give up!*

Conclusions

The preparation of a successful case of need is a skilled task for which most doctors have received no training. The foregoing is necessarily a brief outline of the process. In many cases the establishment of a multi-disciplinary project team to develop the case will be helpful. Assessment of the local situation and identification of influential individuals and groups must come first. Activities related to preparing the document may be as important as the actual content of the finished product. Much remains to be done to accumulate better evidence for the effectiveness of liaison psychiatry services and to develop efficient and practicable methods of measuring outcomes.

Appendix: Check-list of items to consider for inclusion in case of need

- Title of project
- Description of existing service
- Identified health needs of population
- Aims and objectives of new service
- Reasons why needs are not being met by existing services
- Evidence for effectiveness of new service in meeting health needs
- Likely health gains
- Degree of fit with existing strategy and development plans
- Sources of funding
- Implications for other services
- Risks
- Methods of monitoring outcome/audit
- Market research
- Activity, finance and manpower
- Alternative options
- Costs (capital and revenue itemised separately) for each option considered

Acknowledgements

This article was originally based upon a workshop held at the Royal College of Psychiatrists in December 1995. The participants were: Margaret Goose (Nuffield Institute for Health, Leeds), Simon Conway (Deputy Finance Director, West Suffolk NHS Trust), Ben Essex (general practitioner, Sydenham), Jane Davis (Accident and Emergency Service Manager, West Middlesex Hospital), Mike Wear (Director of Public Health, Cornwall) and the following liaison psychiatrists – Francis Creed (Manchester), Eleanor Feldman (Nottingham), Elspeth Guthrie (Manchester), Robert Peveler (Southampton), Amanda Ramirez (London), Michael Sharpe (Edinburgh) and Simon Wessely (London). Comments on the typescript were provided by: Margaret Goose, Ben Essex, Amanda Ramirez, Michael Sharpe, Simon Wessely, Dr Chris Bass and Dr Nick Allen of Southampton and South-West Hampshire Health Authority.

References

DEPARTMENT OF HEALTH (1989) *Caring for People: Community Care in the Next Decade and Beyond.* London: HMSO.

DEPARTMENT OF HEALTH (1994) *Health of the Nation Mental Health Key Area Handbook* (2nd edn). London: HMSO.

DEPARTMENT OF HEALTH (1999) *The National Service Framework for Mental Health.* London: Stationery Office.

HOUSE, A. (1995) Psychiatric disorders, inappropriate health service utilisation and the role of consultation–liaison psychiatry. *Journal of Psychosomatic Research*, **39**, 799–802.

ROYAL COLLEGE OF PHYSICIANS & ROYAL COLLEGE OF PSYCHIATRISTS (1995) *The Psychological Care of Medical Patients: Recognition of Need and Service Provision.* London: Royal College of Physicians/Royal College of Psychiatrists.

ROYAL COLLEGE OF PSYCHIATRISTS (1994) *The General Hospital Management of Adult Deliberate Self-harm: A Consensus Statement on Standards of Service Provision* (CR32) London: Royal College of Psychiatrists.

ROYAL COLLEGE OF SURGEONS (1997) *Report of the Working Party on the Psychological Care of Surgical Patients.* London: Royal College of Surgeons,

SARAVAY, S., STEINBERG, M., WEINSCHEL, B., *et al* (1991) Psychological co-morbidity and length of stay in the general hospital. *American Journal of Psychiatry*, **148**, 324–329.

SAVOCA, E. (1999) Psychiatric co-morbidity and hospital utilisation in the general medical sector. *Psychological Medicine*, **29**, 457–464.

2 Liaison psychiatry in the accident and emergency department

DAVID STORER

This chapter makes the case for an effective psychiatric service to the accident and emergency (A&E) department and suggests that this is best provided by a department of liaison psychiatry. Some details of the clinical service required are also given.

Why does the A&E department require a psychiatric service?

The A&E department is seen by the general public as being the point at which they will receive emergency medical care. Although experienced users of the psychiatric services may be aware of alternative provision, such as community mental health centres, the 'casualty department' is where most members of the public would look for help. In most areas, alternative services are open, at best, during the hours of 9–5, Monday to Friday. General practitioners, in some areas, find that the quickest and easiest way to obtain a psychiatric opinion is to send a patient to the nearest A&E department. If the service users themselves are consulted, they express a preference for a local service that can respond quickly to a crisis at all times (Rogers *et al*, 1993). Johnson & Thornicroft's survey (1995) showed that the A&E department was used in 'normal practice' for assessing psychiatric emergencies in 50% of districts during office hours and in 65% outside office hours. Gater & Goldberg (1991) showed that 16% of 250 consecutive new patients presenting to the psychiatric services in south Manchester arrived via the A&E department. Viewing the problem from an alternative perspective,

30% of A&E attenders can be shown to have psychological/psychiatric problems (Salkovskis *et al*, 1990).

Should the service be provided by liaison psychiatry?

It can be argued that the majority of the psychiatric work seen in an A&E department is, in fact, general psychiatry and therefore should be part of the general service. This model operates successfully in some areas, mainly smaller district general hospitals, particularly where there is a general hospital psychiatric unit. However, there are considerable advantages to a specialised liaison service providing psychiatric cover. Consultants in A&E medicine value being able to contact a psychiatrist who is known to them and who can respond promptly in an emergency (Royal College of Psychiatrists, 1996). One area of clinical practice in which the benefit is seen of close liaison between A&E medicine and liaison psychiatry is in the assessment of deliberate self-harm (DSH). An effective and speedily reactive service to the A&E department at the General Infirmary at Leeds was developed by the department of liaison psychiatry there in the early 1980s (the later development of this department has been described by House, 1994). This service, characterised by excellent working relationships between the staff of both departments, enabled the majority of self-poisoning patients to be admitted to the overnight emergency ward in the A&E department rather than medical wards, which produced a considerable saving in medical bed usage (Table 2.1).

Many A&E departments have such an overnight ward, which can be of considerable value in holding patients whose psychiatric assessment can be more satisfactorily carried out in the morning, when the full multi-disciplinary team is present and other agencies can be more easily contacted. Some departments will not use such a facility for 'psychiatric patients', but if the A&E staff can rely on the prompt availability of a psychiatric team known to them on the

TABLE 2.1
Admissions to general medical beds at Leeds General Infirmary coded as ICD 960–979
(poisoning by drugs)

Year	Total no. of admissions
1977	871
1979	764
1985	177

following day, they show an increased willingness to use the overnight ward for this purpose.

There are great opportunities for joint educational and research work between the two specialities and these are obviously facilitated by close working relationships. Conversely, it is difficult to envisage how this could occur where a succession of different psychiatrists were visiting the A&E department. Apart from the ongoing learning experience for all disciplines in working together on clinical problems, more formal educational activities can be arranged. These can include a regular input from psychiatric staff into the formal educational programme of A&E staff in training and attachments of more senior staff (e.g. specialist registrars) to the psychiatric team.

What should be the model of service?

The provision of a good psychiatric service to a general hospital requires the availability of a strong multi-disciplinary team (Benjamin *et al*, 1994). This is even more the case in relation to the A&E department. Medical, nursing and social work staff are particularly relevant. A&E staff need the consistent availability of psychiatric advice and in an emergency require the prompt attendance of a psychiatrist in their department. The joint report (Royal College of Psychiatrists, 1996) recommended that each general hospital should have a consultant psychiatrist nominated as having a special responsibility for liaising with the A&E department. This may well be the consultant who also takes responsibility for the DSH assessment service.

The Royal College of Psychiatrists also recommends that at least five sessions of consultant liaison psychiatrist time are required to serve the needs of an average-size 'district general hospital' (House & Hodgson, 1994). The duties of this consultant include ensuring the adequate training and supervision of both A&E and psychiatric staff and that a senior clinical opinion is quickly available.

The attachment of specialised psychiatric nurses to an A&E department has been shown to be effective (Storer *et al*, 1987). If the nurse functions as a community psychiatric nurse, then patients can, if necessary, be followed up outside the hospital. Merson *et al* (1992) found that increased follow-up rates and levels of patient satisfaction occurred when emergency attenders received further care at home rather than in an out-patient clinic. However, that study utilised a multi-disciplinary team rather than a community nurse alone. Most departments also find that the employment of psychiatrically trained nurses as part of the A&E staffing improves that department's ability to deal with psychiatric problems. It is unfortunate that, because of changes in nurse education, it is proving increasingly difficult to recruit 'doubly trained' staff. In hospitals with an in-patient psychiatric unit, an alternative is to enhance nurse staffing levels to allow rapid deployment of nurses to the A&E department in an emergency.

Recent enquiries into untoward incidents have drawn wider attention to the need for follow-up of patients leaving hospital before being adequately assessed. A House of Commons (1995) select committee, referring to a case in which a depressed patient left an A&E department in London and committed suicide, made the following recommendation:

"The appointment of a senior mental health liaison nurse is accepted as one method of encouraging close co-operation between mental health services and A&E departments. This recommendation will be brought to the attention of nurse managers of the NHS by Regional Directors of Nursing."

It is not known whether this recommendation has led to any improvement in staffing or services.

There are, of course, alternative models of service provision to that described above. In hospitals that have a general psychiatric unit on site, one can make a case for referrals from the A&E department to be dealt with by the general teams. Less satisfactory is the model whereby psychiatrists on call from the local mental hospital or community unit are called into the A&E department to see cases at the request of the A&E staff. Such services tend to deal with emergency cases only and give rise to problems of supervision of staff and follow-up of patients. Some hospitals remain where a psychiatrist is not available to the A&E staff and patients are dealt with by A&E staff alone or have to be transported to the nearest psychiatric facility to be seen. Johnson & Baderman (1995) reported that 46% of A&E departments in England and Wales do not have psychiatric cover on site outside of working hours.

Merson *et al* (1992) have described an 'early intervention team', which they compared with standard hospital-based care in the management of psychiatric emergencies, 40% of which were referred from the A&E department. However, the patients were seen first and referred on to the team by a duty psychiatrist and the team did not provide a 24-hour service. Such a team can, therefore, be seen as an alternative to a liaison community psychiatric nurse (CPN) rather than a model of a service in itself.

Descriptions of, and comments on, models of service in the USA are given, from a nursing point of view, by Curry (1992) and Snyder (1992).

What is the extent of the problem?

Information on the referral rates from A&E to psychiatry is surprisingly sparse. This may be because, by the nature of A&E as a speciality, information is collected poorly. Referrals are made in emergencies, a note may be made on the 'case card' and the patients are unlikely to be registered in the psychiatric records. A further reason could be that, because services are poorly developed, referrals from A&E have not become a significant part of the system. An analysis of referrals to liaison psychiatry in a large Scottish city reported that "Direct referrals from the Accident & Emergency department are seen by junior medical staff. Such referrals were rare and were not included in the study" (Semple *et al*, 1996).

At Leeds General Infirmary, where an active working relationship between the two departments has existed for many years, referrals from A&E constitute a significant proportion of the working time of medical staff at all levels. The liaison CPN sees approximately 250 A&E attenders per year. At this hospital 2% of A&E attenders present with DSH and a further 1% are given a primary psychiatric diagnosis. Of course, not all of those given a psychiatric diagnosis will be referred to the liaison team and some with other primary diagnoses will be referred.

Bassuk *et al* (1983) reported a comparison of psychiatric emergencies presenting in the emergency room at Beth Israel Hospital, Boston, and at the accident department at Bristol Royal Infirmary. It is interesting and disappointing that most of their findings and conclusions are equally valid today. Over 122 days in Bristol, 163 patients assessed as having overt psychiatric problems other than self-injury presented in Bristol. During the same period, 341 self-injury patients were seen. In a statement prophetic to UK readers, they commented on the situation then in the USA:

> "With increasing medical specialisation, the ascendancy of primary care, and the drift of medical practitioners away from the cities, the numbers of patients using the emergency wards of hospitals in the United States increased dramatically. The progression of de-institutionalisation has further accentuated this trend and has led to a growing number of chronic patients seeking emergency care."

Their conclusion also remains apposite:

> "In both countries, it was not the degree of psychopathology but the lack of an available support network, an inability to engage the patient in the system, and a history of serious chronic maladjustment that led to the majority of 'emergency' visits."

Dunn & Fernando (1989) reported that of 25 651 patients attending an inner London A&E department, 1.8% were allocated a psychiatric diagnosis but 39% of these were DSH patients. Of those with psychiatric diagnoses, 58% were referred to psychiatrists and 240 referrals were seen by psychiatrists over the six-month study period. The authors pointed out that this is likely to be an underestimate and did not discuss whether patients whose primary diagnosis was not psychiatric were referred to psychiatrists. They drew attention to the number of service users using attendance at A&E as a method of self-referral to psychiatrists, which has been seen as a problem in providing an easily accessible psychiatric service to the A&E department.

Crawford & Kohen (1997) analysed referrals to a liaison psychiatry team from an inner London A&E department (Whittington Hospital) over two years. They reported 4815 referrals. Inner London may well have unusual referral patterns, however, as 35% of the patients had been referred to the A&E department by their general practitioner and, surprisingly, 6% by psychiatrists. Ellis & Lewis (1997) reported referrals from another north London hospital and drew attention to the high number of patients with psychiatric needs leaving the A&E department having not been seen by the psychiatric team.

Salkovskis *et al* (1990) carried out a survey of A&E attenders who were not given a psychiatric diagnosis and found that 36% scored above the 'caseness' cut-off point on the General Health Questionnaire or the Hospital Anxiety and Depression Scale. This is a higher proportion than reported in similar surveys of attenders at general practitioners' surgeries. Thirty-two per cent of the patients said that they would like to discuss their worries further with someone. These rates cannot be easily dismissed as merely reflecting the stress of whatever injury or illness led the patients to attend in the first place, as the proportion asking for further help rose to 39% at follow-up one month after attendance. The resource implications of extending a psychiatric service to this group of patients are obvious. However, any proposed interventions need to be carefully evaluated. The same group of authors (Atha *et al*, 1992) carried out a controlled trial of cognitive–behavioural problem solving with patients scoring highly on the above tests, but the results indicated only limited clinical benefits.

The importance of a psychiatric service to the A&E department was illustrated by the presence of a psychiatric member on the influential Accident and Emergency Sub-group of the London Implementation Group, which was responsible for making the recommendations that led to the reshaping of acute hospital services in London.

What resources are required to provide the service?

In order that referrals to the psychiatric team can be assessed safely and effectively, at least one satisfactory interview room is required in the A&E department. Ideally, this room should be specifically for psychiatric use but this may not be possible in small departments. The room needs to be situated centrally enough to be within sight and hearing of A&E staff; it should not be isolated in an inaccessible part of the department nor at the end of a corridor. It should be well lit, preferably by daylight and in a good state of decoration. The decor should be in quiet, calming colours and the room should be furnished with comfortable easy chairs and a coffee table rather than a desk. In the interests of safety the room should have more than one, outwardly opening, door. There should be an observation window so that the occupants can be seen from outside. There should be an easily accessible 'panic button' with connection to the staff area nearby. No furniture or fittings should be usable as weapons. Ideally, a closed-circuit television security system should be in operation.

The increasing problem of acute intoxication with drugs has been recognised in some centres by the provision of a dedicated 'detoxification room', allowing patients to be treated in a safe, secure place over several hours.

What are the staffing implications?

Reference to the need for a consultant to take overall responsibility for the service to the A&E department has been made above. The sessional commitment required to carry this out will depend on the workload from the department in question and also on the medical and non-medical support available. Where doctors in training are allocated to the liaison team, they will be involved in providing the service but will still require the allocation of consultant time for the provision of supervision. In some hospitals a full-time or part-time doctor in a non-training grade (e.g. associate specialist or staff grade) may be employed to provide the clinical service, but, again, some level of consultant supervision is required.

Many A&E departments employ nurses who are psychiatrically trained. This can be a great asset in the understanding of patients presenting with psychiatric problems and also aids communication with the psychiatric team. Recent changes in nurse training are leading to a decreasing number of 'doubly qualified' nurses, so such nurses are becoming more difficult to recruit and retain. The attachment of a CPN to the A&E department has been described earlier. The CPN can be used to follow-up patients who have caused concern to the A&E staff but who would not remain in the department to be seen by the psychiatric team. The CPN may also be involved in interventions with specific patient groups. For example, individual protocols may be devised for frequent attenders at the A&E department so that they can be handled consistently rather than repeated assessments being carried out by different psychiatrists. The CPN is ideally placed to provide the consistency and continuity required by such protocols. A base in the psychiatric department and a daily presence in the A&E department enables the CPN to be a key link between the departments.

It has been suggested (Royal College of Psychiatrists, 1996) that the nurse staffing of psychiatric units in general hospitals should be enhanced to allow "the rapid deployment of psychiatric nurses into the A&E department when required, particularly in emergency situations". Similarly, such enhancement of staffing can provide a capability to provide psychiatric nursing support and expertise to the non-psychiatric wards in the hospital. Unfortunately, however, nurse managements are tending to reduce ward staffing levels to the bare minimum (or below!) and such flexibility is becoming increasingly difficult to achieve.

Most A&E departments have an attached social worker who may, or may not, have the training, confidence and/or inclination to be involved with mental health problems. It is necessary to agree a system whereby an approved social worker can be rapidly available for Mental Health Act purposes.

The service for the assessment of DSH patients needs to be closely linked to the A&E department. In most hospitals the liaison psychiatry team will be responsible for both services. If there is a specialist multidisciplinary team for the assessment and follow-up of DSH cases it needs to be based in, or have close links with, the A&E department. Some of these teams also offer a 'crisis intervention' service to the A&E department.

What are the educational needs and opportunities?

Close cooperative working between the specialities of liaison psychiatry and A&E medicine can provide fruitful opportunities for education, research and audit.

The most valuable form of education is that of 'on the job learning', which is most productive when two teams who are accustomed to working together can learn from each other. This relatively informal style of learning should be allied to formal educational occasions and to regular supervision.

As far as medical staff are concerned, such a working pattern is a good model for undergraduates to see, and for postgraduates in both specialities, as well as those undergoing basic professional education in psychiatry, to be involved in. It is also a relevant area for those training for a career in general practice. A&E medicine is a well organised speciality as far as postgraduate medical education is concerned and most departments have an in-house educational programme for their senior house officers. It is important for psychiatrists to be involved in this teaching programme at an early stage so that new senior house officers have some knowledge of the diagnostic principles of psychiatry, how and when to refer to the psychiatric team and the initial management of psychiatric emergencies. Those doctors intending to become consultants in A&E medicine should have a longer exposure to liaison psychiatry and in some regional higher training schemes in England specialist registrars are seconded to departments of liaison psychiatry for up to a month at a time.

Psychiatric trainees will gain experience in this field during their attachments to liaison psychiatry. In some hospitals, specific attachments of psychiatrists in higher training to A&E departments have been arranged so that a specialist registrar will be responsible, under consultant direction, for organising, and to some extent providing, the psychiatric input.

Similar educational opportunities exist for other disciplines, in particular nursing. This is an ideal liaison situation for learning from other disciplines through working together. Formal educational activities such as multi-disciplinary case conferences could occur and would be valuable but are difficult to organise.

Examples of research and clinical audit are sparse in the literature, which is disappointing as there is considerable potential for both (Atha *et al*, 1989). Some of the publications in the area have been discussed earlier. An audit of DSH services in A&E has been described by Hughes *et al* (1998).

What are the difficulties?

Many of the practical day-to-day difficulties arise because of the diversities of clinical problems presenting in the A&E department and the frequent lack of information outside of that immediately obtainable from history taking and examination. The diversity of presentation, apart from presenting difficulties, is also one of the stimulating challenges presented to the psychiatrist in this work. The gathering of supporting information can often be laborious and frustrating. Any previous psychiatric records may well be in another hospital or even another part of the country. If the patient is accompanied then obviously more information is obtainable but often the telephone has to be an essential part of the psychiatrist's assessment equipment.

Accident and emergency staff are frequently concerned about the legal aspects of assessing and treating psychiatric patients. A common scenario is that of a clearly disturbed individual who may also be physically ill or suffering from the effects of DSH who refuses treatment. Psychiatrists can sometimes be placed under pressure to use the Mental Health Act in order to 'legitimise' treatment without the patient's consent. A&E staff are sometimes reluctant to administer treatment under common law and find it hard to appreciate that 'sectioning' a patient does not give them additional rights to administer medical treatments without consent. In some hospitals, security staff are unwilling to assist in restraining patients and apply inappropriate pressure for the Mental Health Act to be used. These medico-legal issues are dealt with in more detail in Chapter 6.

In some areas of the UK, the A&E department is regarded as a place of safety under section 136 of the Act. Most consultants in A&E medicine are strongly opposed to this, as they believe that such use of their department is inappropriate and they do not have the facilities to provide the appropriate assessment. It is doubtful whether liaison psychiatry is an appropriate speciality to take the leading role in such assessments. In most areas the prompt attendance of a senior psychiatrist at a police station is regarded as a more satisfactory way of dealing with section 136.

Difficulties familiar to liaison psychiatrists in other areas of their work are pertinent to the A&E service, in particular the related questions of resources and relations with other psychiatric services. Lloyd (1996) has discussed the difficulties of obtaining resources for psychiatry in the general hospital in the era of 'community psychiatry' and Wessely (1996) has referred to the 'New Alienists'. Lloyd strongly advocates that liaison psychiatrists should be employed by acute trusts. Kessel (1996) presents the opposing view but repeats the popular misconception of liaison psychiatry as an esoteric 'optional extra', separate from the mainstream of psychiatry. A short time accompanying a psychiatrist in A&E should dispel this view and those who regard general hospitals as not part of the community may care to work a Friday or Saturday evening shift in an inner-city casualty department.

Good working relationships and clear delineation of responsibilities need to be established with the other sub-specialities within psychiatry. As far as general psychiatry is concerned, it is necessary to be able to arrange emergency admission if necessary, to be able to request longer-term community follow-up if this is more appropriate than the shorter-term involvement of liaison staff and also to communicate rapidly with general teams when their existing patients appear at the A&E department (around 30% of psychiatric referrals from A&E at Leeds General Infirmary). Similar relationships are required with old age psychiatry but some psychiatrists for the elderly prefer to see referrals over the age of 65 from A&E themselves if they are based in the general hospital. Similarly, child and adolescent psychiatrists will normally see A&E attenders who are still at school. A procedure needs to be agreed with the learning disabilities service for the assessment of the occasional mentally handicapped person attending A&E. Drug and alcohol problems are, of course, exceedingly common in A&E (Ghodse *et al*, 1981) and close liaison with the local substance misuse service is essential. Wylie *et al* (1996) have suggested having an addictions CPN with special responsibilities to the general hospital.

Negotiating for resources

This chapter is intended to contain information useful in the preparation of a 'business case' for a liaison service. In most hospitals there is ready support for such a service from the staff and management of the A&E department itself. However, such support may well not be accompanied by resources. None the less, in the current 'internal market' A&E services are usually funded by 'block contracts' and it may be possible to include the liaison service in such a contract as an 'added value' item. This is likely to be the most fruitful course if the liaison psychiatry service is part of the acute trust. However, if all psychiatric services are part of a community trust, the inclusion of the service to A&E in the overall contract for emergency psychiatric cover may be a better option.

Conclusions

The difficulties and frustrations of providing a psychiatric service to the A&E department have been described but an attempt has also been made to convey the challenge and even excitement of working with colleagues in the most acute of specialities. The opportunities for liaison not only with specialists in A&E medicine but also with our colleagues in other psychiatric sub-specialities and in general medical practice are also stimulating. The valuable multi-disciplinary educational opportunities are an additional benefit of this branch of liaison psychiatry.

References

ATHA, C., SALKOVSKIS, P. M. & STORER, D. (1989) Accident and emergency: more questions than answers. *Nursing Times*, **85**, 28–31.

—, — & — (1992) Cognitive–behavioural problem solving in the treatment of patients attending a medical emergency department: a controlled trial. *Journal of Psychosomatic Research*, **30**, 299–307.

BASSUK, E. L., WINTER, R. & APSLER, R. (1983) Cross-cultural comparison of British and American psychiatric emergencies. *American Journal of Psychiatry*, **140**, 180–184.

BENJAMIN, S., HOUSE, A. & JENKINS, P. (eds) (1994) *Liaison Psychiatry. Defining Needs and Planning Services*. London: Gaskell.

CRAWFORD, M. J. & KOHEN, D. (1997) Urgent psychiatric assessment in an inner-city A&E department. *Psychiatric Bulletin*, **21**, 625–626.

CURRY, J. (1992) Care of psychiatric patients in the emergency department. *Journal of Emergency Nursing*, **29**, 396–407.

DUNN, J. & FERNANDO, R. (1989) Psychiatric presentations to an accident and emergency department. *Psychiatric Bulletin*, **13**, 672–674.

ELLIS, D. & LEWIS, S. (1997) Psychiatric presentations to an A&E department. *Psychiatric Bulletin*, **21**, 627–630.

GATER, R. & GOLDBERG, D. (1991) Pathways to psychiatric care in south Manchester. *British Journal of Psychiatry*, **159**, 90–96.

GHODSE, A. H., Edwards, G., Stapleton, J., *et al* (1981) Drug related problems in London accident and emergency departments. *Lancet*, *i*, 859–862.

HOUSE, A. (1994) Liaison psychiatry in a large teaching hospital, the service at Leeds General Infirmary. In *Liaison Psychiatry. Defining Needs and Planning Services* (eds S. Benjamin, A. House & P. Jenkins), pp. 58–64. London: Gaskell.

— & Hodgson, G. (1994) Estimating needs and meeting demands. In *Liaison Psychiatry. Defining Needs and Planning Services* (eds S. Benjamin, A. House & P. Jenkins), pp. 3–15. London: Gaskell.

HOUSE OF COMMONS (1995) *Government Response to the Second Report from the Select Committee on the Parliamentary Commission for Administration, Sessions 1994–95 on the Report of the Health Service Commissions for 1993–94*. London: HMSO.

HUGHES, T., HAMPSHAW, S., RENVOIZE, E., *et al* (1998) General hospital services for those who carry out deliberate self-harm. *Psychiatric Bulletin*, **22**, 88–91.

JOHNSON, S. & BADERMAN, H. (1995) Psychiatric emergencies in the casualty department. In *Emergency Mental Health Services in the Community* (eds M. Phelan, G. Strathdee & G. Thornicroft), pp. 213–232. Cambridge: Cambridge University Press.

— & Thornicroft, G. (1995) Emergency psychiatric services in England and Wales. *British Medical Journal*, **311**, 287–288.

KESSEL, N. (1996) Should we buy liaison psychiatry? *Journal of the Royal Society of Medicine*, **89**, 481–482.

LLOYD, G.G. (1996) A sense of proportion: the place of psychiatry in medicine. *Journal of the Royal Society of Medicine*, **89**, 563–567.

MERSON, S., TYRER, P., ONYETT, S., *et al* (1992) Early intervention in psychiatric emergencies: a controlled clinical trial. *Lancet*, **339**, 1311–1314.

ROGERS, A., PILGRIM, D. & LACEY, R. (1993) *Experiencing Psychiatry*. London: Macmillan.

ROYAL COLLEGE OF PSYCHIATRISTS (1996) *Psychiatric Services to Accident and Emergency Departments. Report of a Joint Working Party of the Royal College of Psychiatrists and the British Association for Accident and Emergency Medicine* (CR43). London: Royal College of Psychiatrists.

SALKOVSKIS, P. M., STORER, D., ATHA, C., *et al* (1990) Psychiatric morbidity in an accident and emergency department. *British Journal of Psychiatry*, **156**, 483–487.

SEMPLE, M., BROWN, D. & IRVINE, E. (1996) Liaison psychiatry in detection and management of mental illness. *Psychiatric Bulletin*, **20**, 466–469.

SNYDER, J. (1992) Specialised services for psychiatric patients in the emergency department. *Journal of Emergency Nursing*, **18**, 535–536.

STORER, D., WHITWORTH, R., SALKOVSKIS, P., *et al* (1987) Community psychiatric nursing intervention in an accident and emergency department: a clinical pilot study. *Journal of Advanced Nursing*, **12**, 215–222.

WESSELY, S. (1996) The rise of counselling and the return of alienism. *British Medical Journal*, **313**, 158–160.

WYLIE, K., HOUSE, A., STORER, D., *et al* (1996) Deliberate self-harm and substance dependence: the management of patients seen in the general hospital. *Journal of Mental Health Administration*, **23**, 246–251.

3 Services for deliberate self-harm patients

NAVNEET KAPUR and DAVID OWENS

If, as Sakinofsky & Roberts (1990) argue, and perhaps many others suspect, psychosocial programmes of intervention following deliberate self-harm have failed, why should health commissioners commit precious resources to the purchase of any kind of service for assessment or intervention? This chapter sets out some answers to this conundrum.

The need for assessment and treatment services for self-harm patients

Deliberate self-harm is a persistently important public health problem, usually said to account for more than 100 000 hospital admissions in England and Wales each year. This estimate is likely to be far lower than the true number of episodes, for two reasons. First, many of those who harm themselves never present to hospital (Kennedy et al, 1974). Second, there is a trend towards discharge of deliberate self-harm patients directly from accident and emergency departments (Owens, 1990), and a recent estimate of hospital *attendances* is around 140 000 in England and Wales each year (Hawton et al, 1997).

Deliberate self-harm has serious sequelae: 1% of patients go on to kill themselves in the year following the self-harm episode (Hawton & Fagg, 1988) – a 100-fold increase in baseline risk – and an estimated 10% eventually complete suicide (Nordentoft et al, 1993). Repetition has been found to be between 10% and 30% per annum – most often around 12–15%. In England and Wales these outcome rates mean that there may be 1000–1500 suicides (a quarter or more of the annual total of suicides) and perhaps 15 000 non-fatal episodes each year that may be amenable to secondary prevention following a non-fatal self-harm episode. Recent policy initiatives, such as *The Health of the Nation* in England, have drawn attention to efforts to reduce suicide rates; effective help for deliberate self-harm patients may make a significant contribution towards meeting the targets set.

Although it is widely held that psychosocial intervention following self-harm has no impact, research evidence suggests that services for deliberate self-harm can be effective. Of the five controlled trials of psychosocial interventions for adult self-harm patients in the UK, all showed benefit in terms of social adjustment, satisfaction with services or improved affective symptoms (Owens & House, 1994). Four of the five studies also showed a reduced repetition rate. Unfortunately, the sample size in each of these studies was too small for the potentially important reductions in repetition rate to reach statistical significance. A systematic review of the world literature of clinical trials of psychosocial and pharmacological treatments in preventing repetition has recently been undertaken (Hawton *et al*, 1998), using the protocols for the Cochrane Collaboration. It concludes that at present there is insufficient evidence to indicate the most effective form of treatment for patients who deliberately harm themselves. The authors suggest that further research is urgently needed. The dilemma is that because of the scale and seriousness of the problem we can see the need to provide effective deliberate self-harm services but cannot be at all sure of what approaches are most worthwhile until we have research findings from much larger studies.

The inconsistency of current service provision

The history of planned services for deliberate self-harm begins with the brief guidance issued to hospitals by the Minister of Health when attempted suicide ceased to be unlawful in 1961; inconsistencies in provision have been a feature ever since. Blake & Mitchell (1978) audited the management of self-poisoning by 10 psychiatric teams responsible for assessments in two hospitals in Nottingham and found wide differences in their decisions. For instance, further follow-up was arranged for almost all patients by one team but for less than half by another. More recently, reported rates of referral for psychiatric care have ranged between 21% (Hawton & Catalan, 1987) and 76% (Hamer *et al*, 1991). Similarly, there is a great discrepancy between proportions discharged directly from accident and emergency departments without formal psychiatric assessment: figures from our recent study of hospitals in Leeds, Nottingham, Leicester and Manchester show discharge rates ranging from 18% to 76% (Kapur *et al*, 1998). Part of the reason for these variations is a lack of agreement about the nature of proper clinical management. In an unpublished 1991 study, Renvoize & Storer found that less than half of the health districts in the Yorkshire health region had written guidelines on the management of deliberate self-harm, or a named consultant psychiatrist with a responsibility for the service. Hawton & James (1995) found that only five of the nine hospitals they surveyed in the Oxford region had written guidelines in place.

In 1994, the Royal College of Psychiatrists sought to clarify matters by producing a consensus statement on the standards of service provision for adult deliberate self-harm in the general hospital. It set out recommendations for organisation of services and patient management, more wide-ranging and detailed than the official guidelines of 10 years before (Department of Health and Social Security, 1984), and is essential reading for anyone involved in provision of deliberate self-harm services in the UK.

Planning a self-harm service

The first priority following an episode of deliberate self-harm is to ensure that the individual's physical condition is thoroughly assessed and appropriately managed. Thereafter, a psychosocial assessment needs to be carried out in order to identify and do something for those at high risk of suicide and those with significant mental health problems. Research suggests that as many as 40% of self-harm patients may be suffering from an affective disorder and 30% may have a serious problem with alcohol misuse (Ennis *et al*, 1989). The service also needs to be able to offer social and psychological interventions for the range of problems commonly encountered among deliberate self-harm patients.

Setting up a planning group

Setting up a planning group for deliberate self-harm services, made up of people from different strands of the health service, is a first step towards rational planning. This group might include an accident and emergency consultant, psychiatric consultant, accident and emergency nurse, psychiatric nurse, social worker, senior manager, general practitioner and a representative of the purchasers. Inclusion of an information officer would help with the necessary audit and service monitoring.

Determining the current situation

Before planning a new service or altering existing services, the planning group should consider the demographic characteristics, specific needs and service implications of the catchment population – for instance, the prevalence of those whose first language is not English, or of those who are elderly. It also needs to establish what are the activities of the existing self-harm service (if any), because they may offer clues regarding the need for change. For example, in some places there are well structured arrangements in place for the assessment and subsequent care of patients admitted to medical wards, with referral of suitable patients to sector community mental health teams, but little attention to an equally large number of patients discharged directly from accident and emergency departments. It is essential to have a clear picture of the number (and proportions) of patients attending, admitted, assessed and treated, in order to set up the most appropriate training, supervision and deployment of staff.

Planning the care in various settings

Deliberate self-harm services need to be provided in three broad areas: in accident and emergency departments, on in-patient wards and in the community. We have made a distinction between assessment and management by *non-specialists* (usually physicians and general nurses, in accident and emergency departments and on in-patient wards) and *specialists* (usually mental health staff). Each of these areas is discussed under separate headings below.

Non-specialist services in accident and emergency departments

In most hospitals one of the first tasks for the planning group will be to review the admissions policy for deliberate self-harm. In our own hospital it is policy that all self-harm patients are admitted, regardless of the medical seriousness of the act. This has several practical advantages: it makes subsequent psychosocial assessment much easier, makes it possible to obtain information from informants, allows temporary respite, provides an opportunity for positive care by nursing staff and allows time to organise social interventions. In a great many hospitals, however, the state of play is quite different.

The current official guidelines on the management of deliberate self-harm (Department of Health and Social Security, 1984) acknowledge that general practitioners will manage some cases at home and that some patients will be discharged from accident and emergency care without seeing a psychiatrist. Since the early 1980s, increased pressure on medical beds and on costs has meant that ever greater numbers of patients are discharged directly from an accident and emergency department without a psychiatric assessment (Owens, 1990). Our recent descriptive study carried out in four centres across the UK suggested that from some accident and emergency departments as many as 75% of those attending after self-harm are discharged (Kapur *et al*, 1998). Consequently, accident and emergency management of deliberate self-harm is more important now than ever.

Initial assessment

The accident and emergency management of deliberate self-harm begins with triage. The nurse needs to make a preliminary assessment of the patient's physical condition, the degree of distress and the likelihood that the patient will remain in the department to see the accident and emergency doctor, and take any necessary action. After their initial physical condition has been adequately attended to, some patients will be admitted to the medical in-patient unit. For others there will be plans for them to return home. If so, a comprehensive psychosocial assessment needs to be carried out. Depending on local policy and the time of day, this task may be the responsibility of the designated deliberate self-harm team or duty psychiatrist. But, in practice, many of those who go home from accident and emergency departments receive psychosocial assessment only by non-specialist accident and emergency medical and nursing staff. This in itself may not be a major cause for concern, as there is some tentative evidence that accident and emergency staff can screen self-harm patients adequately (Gardner *et al*, 1982; Waterhouse & Platt, 1990; Owens *et al*, 1991). However, it does mean that training, supervision and sufficient time for the task of assessment become essential prerequisites for accident and emergency medical and nursing staff who carry out such work.

Advice, supervision and referring on

The day-to-day supervision of psychosocial assessments can properly be undertaken only by senior staff who have had some training in psychiatry or another appropriate mental health discipline. Some recently trained accident and emergency consultants are likely to have gained the necessary experience from a substantial placement in psychiatry during their training. If not, other supervisors need to be identified – in many cases the consultant psychiatrist with responsibility for accident and emergency referrals.

Accident and emergency staff need ready telephone access to a psychiatrist or member of the deliberate self-harm team and on occasions face-to-face contact. Some busy accident and emergency departments have deployed a senior nurse who has psychiatric training, or found room for a liaison psychiatrist to be attached to the department. In our own hospital's accident and emergency department we have an attached community psychiatric nurse, who can carry out home visits as well as work in the department; accident and emergency staff can refer patients who have left the hospital without a full assessment.

Training

If an accident and emergency department regularly discharges deliberate self-harm patients, training for new staff needs to be arranged soon after they join the department – perhaps as part of an induction programme. At its completion, each person should be able to carry out a systematic psychosocial assessment in an agreed and probably standardised format, to include an assessment of suicide risk, perhaps using one of the scales that are widely available (Kreitman & Foster, 1991). The training should impart a basic understanding of when duty of care requires the doctor to hold and treat people against their will and when to seek psychiatric advice about use of the Mental Health Act. In addition, staff need to be aware of the local facilities and services that are in place. The Royal College consensus statement (1994) suggests that the local self-harm planning group can improve training for and assessment by non-specialist staff by producing a pre-printed check-list (see Appendix). This would also help with monitoring standards.

Communication

Communication between professionals about recent self-harm is often less than adequate. If someone attends and leaves the accident and emergency department after an episode of self-harm, a designated staff member should rapidly inform the general practitioner, the patient's psychiatric team (if applicable) and any other agencies involved, by telephone if urgency warrants it. In all cases a letter should be forwarded to the general practitioner within a few days.

Facilities

The environment in which assessments are conducted should be adequate. The interview should be carried out in a setting that is private and likely to be reasonably free from interruption. Many accident and emergency departments prefer to use a designated room for this purpose. It is important that such rooms are suitably sited, not far from well staffed areas, and have security systems for the safety of staff. There will be occasions when routine assessments cannot be carried out in such a room, for example if the patient is unduly threatening. At such times more than one member of staff may need to be present at the psychosocial assessment and it may promote safety if hospital security staff are at hand during the interview.

Non-specialist services on in-patient wards

In our hospital, audit suggests that most of those admitted as medical (or, less often, surgical) in-patients after deliberate self-harm receive specialist assessments. However, in most hospitals it is *assumed* that nearly all admitted patients are referred, but this is rarely checked. In practice, there may well be a substantial proportion of in-patients who discharge themselves or refuse or are not offered assessment. A study in one hospital some years ago (Collier *et al*, 1976) found that only 43% of admitted self-harm patients were referred for psychosocial assessment.

It is axiomatic that where patients are appropriately discharged directly from the accident and emergency department because of their low risk of repetition or suicide, then the remainder, admitted to the wards, represent a high-risk group with a greater concentration of psychiatric morbidity. The national increase in the proportion of patients discharged from accident and emergency care thereby renders the assessment of in-patients an increasingly complex task (Owens, 1990).

Training, supervision and facilities

In a clinical trial, physicians proved capable of making satisfactory psychosocial assessments of self-harm in-patients in a setting where training, supervision and access to specialist back-up were provided (Gardner *et al*, 1977). However, there is no evidence, and it seems improbable, that untrained and unsupervised physicians and surgeons can safely make psychosocial assessments. As with other aspects of care, psychosocial management is the responsibility of the whole medical and nursing team and should not be left to an unsupervised pre-registration house officer. If medical or surgical teams intend to undertake their own psychosocial assessments, they will need the kind of training and supervision referred to above in relation to accident and emergency staff and, similarly, the ward-based medical staff will need to have a basic understanding of when they can and cannot treat patients against their will. Whoever undertakes the psychosocial assessment should take responsibility for informing the general practitioner and any other relevant professionals about a patient's admission.

Interview facilities on wards should be adequate and the planning group may wish to facilitate systematic assessments by producing a check-list of the type described above (see Appendix). In many hospitals, patients who have harmed themselves are admitted to a designated short-stay or assessment ward associated with the accident and emergency department. This arrangement enables staff on that ward, especially where some of them have psychiatric training, to acquire expertise, and it simplifies the referral process to the specialist teams.

Policy for assessment

In some hospitals there may be agreement between physicians and psychiatrists that suitably trained and supervised physicians are to undertake psychosocial assessments of in-patients and will refer to specialists only those patients deemed to be at high risk of further self-harm. If so, there should be regular meetings between physicians and the specialist self-harm team or senior psychiatrist to ensure that the service runs smoothly and to provide for supervision. Policies and procedures regarding referral can thereby be kept under review. For example, some target groups of patients may be exceptions. For instance, we think that patients who are over 65 years of age, those who are still at school and those with a learning disability should normally be referred to specialist services (see below).

Specialist services for deliberate self-harm

Specialist services will be involved in *consultation* work, assessing patients who have been referred by the hospital staff from the accident and emergency department and medical wards following episodes of deliberate self-harm. They are also likely to work in a *liaison* style, working closely with the medical or nursing team, perhaps attending ward rounds, discussing patients' needs and supervising and supporting staff. Some specialist teams deal exclusively with deliberate self-harm while others have a wider function in liaison and consultation. The main advantage of a dedicated self-harm service is that assessments are not relegated to extra tasks squeezed in at the end of a long day. On the other hand, working exclusively with deliberate self-harm is extremely demanding and can lead to demoralisation and burnout, especially if there is inadequate staff support.

Deliberate self-harm teams or psychiatrists?

There is evidence that adequate psychosocial assessments of self-harm patients can be made by staff other than psychiatrists, such as social workers (Gibbons *et al*, 1978; Newson-Smith & Hirsch, 1979) and psychiatric nurses (Catalan *et al*, 1980). On the other hand, if a large proportion of self-harm patients suffer from psychiatric disorder (estimates range from 10% to 60%), is assessment by a psychiatrist indispensable? The solution to this dilemma is to adopt a multi-disciplinary team approach to the assessment of deliberate self-harm. This has several advantages: the range of available interventions is increased, a wide range of skills can be shared and expertise can develop. Not least, the team approach helps to maintain morale, which is particularly important as work brings about many difficult encounters and decisions. Such a team may include psychiatric nurses, social workers and psychiatrists. Specialists such as clinical psychologists and occupational therapists may also contribute, although in practice this is rare. Suitable leadership and clinical supervision depend on local circumstances but may be provided by the consultant psychiatrist with responsibility for deliberate self-harm services. It is our view, and that of the Royal College of Psychiatrists (1994), that this team approach is to be preferred, although it may not be feasible in small districts, particularly in rural areas. The prevalence of multi-disciplinary deliberate self-harm services seems to be increasing, perhaps in part as a consequence of pressures to reduce the workload and hours of work of junior doctors.

If trainee psychiatrists are properly to assess patients who have carried out deliberate self-harm, this part of their work needs to be sensibly scheduled and not, as is often the case, squeezed in whenever existing duties allow. Unfortunately, in many hospitals, junior psychiatrists carry out assessments on a rota basis with nominal supervision from the on-call psychiatric specialist registrar or consultant, whose advice is available only if sought. Where we work, much more satisfactory supervision is provided by daily face-to-face meetings between the trainees undertaking assessments and someone from a rota of specialist registrars and consultants in liaison psychiatry.

There are persuasive arguments for adopting a liaison style of service rather than having a 'team of the day' (House & Hodgson, 1994): administrative efficiency and speed of response are increased, the consistency of management decisions is improved and specific training and educational opportunities are provided. Too often this work is regarded as an additional and onerous chore. In addition, staff build up a knowledge of suitable sources of statutory and voluntary agency help for the problems that beset self-harm patients, such as debt, legal problems and relationship difficulties. However, for such a system to work there needs to be adequate support from the general psychiatric services out of hours, at weekends and over holidays.

Training and supervision

The Royal College of Psychiatrists (1994) has set out standards for training and supervision. Someone new to the assessment of deliberate self-harm should undertake it under direct supervision until judged competent. In at least five cases the supervisor should make face-to-face contact with the patient being assessed. New staff should be pointed towards relevant literature, for example that concerning the well established risk factors associated with subsequent suicide or further self-harm (Williams & Morgan, 1994) and the statutory and voluntary sources of help for the problems commonly encountered by self-harm patients.

During the first six months of self-harm assessments, every case should be supervised to some extent. The patient's management should be discussed in detail with the designated supervisor. Emergency assessments out of hours also need to be discussed; in most hospitals this supervision will probably be provided by the on-call specialist registrar or consultant. After the first six months, every case need not be discussed in detail. As greater experience is acquired, the trainee can make an informed choice about when to discuss patient management with a more senior person.

Assessment or intervention?

In many hospitals the deliberate self-harm service provides only assessment and consultations and advice to medical staff and patients in the accident and emergency department and on in-patient wards; any follow-up required is supposed to be provided by the sector psychiatric team, the general practitioner or other locally available services. However, hard-pressed general practitioners may not act on recommendations arising from the self-harm assessment (Hawton *et al*, 1987) and non-attendance rates for follow-up are high (Owens *et al*, 1991). In addition there is the dilemma of which patients to refer to the psychiatric services: just those with a formal psychiatric disorder, or patients with psychosocial problems who may well be helped by brief psychological treatment? One of the advantages of the team approach to deliberate self-harm is that it is possible to provide a comprehensive service, including intervention. Compliance with any therapy is likely to benefit from continuity resulting from the same person carrying out both the initial assessment and subsequent follow-up (Moller, 1989), and from home visits (Hawton *et al*, 1981). Often, repetition of self-harm happens quickly; in a recent study of those who repeated within a year of an index episode, we found the median time to repetition was just 12 weeks (Gilbody *et al*, 1997). Any follow-up usually needs to be rapid and so is more easily provided by a specialist team.

What type of psychosocial intervention should the team provide? Its multi-disciplinary nature will usually allow for a range of options. There is increasing interest in interventions that are cognitively based, concentrate on interpersonal relationships, or are family or systems based. *Problem-solving* therapy is a brief, problem-oriented, cognitively based treatment that is easily taught. Small controlled clinical trials have suggested that it is effective following deliberate self-harm (Salkovskis *et al*, 1990; McLeavy *et al*, 1994), although, as discussed above, sample sizes were too small to show an effect on repetition rates. Hawton & Kirk (1989) provide a useful introduction to problem-solving therapy. From a preliminary study (Morgan *et al*, 1993) it seems that giving first-time self-harm patients written guidance on how to gain access to psychiatric help at times of crises may also be of benefit.

Operational policies

Referral policies need to be agreed by the planning group and the system for referring patients should be clearly understood by the referrer, any clerical staff who pass on the details of referrals, and the deliberate self-harm team. It has been suggested that an urgent request for consultation, either on the wards or in the accident and emergency department, should result in a member of the deliberate self-harm team or duty psychiatrist attending within one hour (Royal College of Psychiatrists, 1994). Non-urgent cases should be seen on the same working day if the referral is made in the first part of the morning or within 24 hours if the referral comes later in the day. Clear policies also need to be drawn up about supervision, clinical responsibility and communication with the general practitioner and other professionals involved (see above).

Community services for deliberate self-harm

Some people do not come to the attention of mental health or specialist self-harm services after they have harmed themselves. Many are seen by a general practitioner and do not attend hospital

(Kennedy *et al*, 1974). Others have no contact with specialist services during or after their attendance at hospital (Owens *et al*, 1991). Community services for deliberate self-harm are likely to be of benefit to some from each of these groups. Such a service could be co-ordinated by either the specialist service or the sector team and may take the form of a drop-in clinic or a community nurse visiting people at home. Organisations from the voluntary and statutory sectors also have an important role to play in providing services such as crisis counselling, in raising public awareness and in liaison with the local self-harm planning group. In practice, though, the growth of community provision in general mental health care has unfortunately not been paralleled by similar development of community care for deliberate self-harm patients.

Special services for special groups

Those over 65 years of age who harm themselves often have very different problems from younger patients; for example, they have a higher prevalence of mood disorder and physical illness (Dennis & Lindesay, 1995). Similarly, the assessment and management of school-age children and those with a learning disability require specific skills that are unlikely to be provided with uniform quality by a general deliberate self-harm team, still less a duty rota self-harm assessment system. For that reason all such patients should, in the view of the Royal College of Psychiatrists (1994), be assessed by the appropriate specialist team.

Even when the above groups are excluded, self-harm patients do not form a homogeneous population. It is likely that different interventions will benefit different subgroups; we should look towards targeting specific interventions at specific groups, such as those who repeat self-harm, those who cut themselves and those with drug or alcohol problems (House *et al*, 1992). Two treatments have been shown to be effective for people who repeatedly harm themselves: problem-solving treatment (Salkovskis *et al*, 1990) and dialectical behaviour therapy (Linehan *et al*, 1993). There is very little robust evidence of benefits for other subgroups.

Audit and service monitoring

Although it would plainly be good practice for a hospital to determine and monitor trends in outcome following hospital attendance as a result of deliberate self-harm, most hospitals have not yet taken the rudimentary step of recording the number and demographic characteristics of attenders and what arrangements are made for them once they leave. How many attend the accident and emergency department? What proportion is discharged from there? Which of them receive a specialist assessment? What proportion is transferred from the general hospital to psychiatric wards? A disconcerting finding in Hawton & James's (1995) survey, carried out after publication of the Royal College guidelines, was that only four out of nine hospitals surveyed could supply information on the proportion of their deliberate self-harm patients discharged directly from the accident and emergency department.

The Royal College statement includes many readily definable standards for facilities, policies and clinical practice that are amenable to audit. Case note review should be carried out to determine the standard of service in the accident and emergency department and on the wards. Discharge and after-care arrangements should also be monitored. It is expecting a lot for individual hospitals to undertake regular monitoring of repetition and subsequent suicide rates; such work is more akin to that required for a research project. However, it may be that the new arrangements for the national confidential enquiry into suicides, based in Manchester, will allow for cross-checking of names of deliberate self-harm attenders and those who have died by suicide (or probable suicide).

Conclusions

We have a responsibility to ensure that all deliberate self-harm patients are properly assessed and directed towards any appropriate further care. Around the country consistent and comprehensive services should be in place. Published guidelines from the Royal College of Psychiatrists (1994) are available to help with this process. A good first step would be to set up cross-disciplinary self-harm planning groups in each hospital or district. Accurate information on current services will be needed before rational planning can direct the available resources. In particular, those planning the service need to know about the numbers and proportions of patients attending and leaving accident and emergency care. Multi-disciplinary deliberate self-harm teams are becoming an increasingly popular means of service provision and have several advantages over older models of working. Further research is urgently needed to identify what interventions are effective and which of these benefit specific subgroups of patients. Only through training, supervision, regular audit and frequent service monitoring can we ensure that the minimum acceptable standards are achieved and maintained. Finally, it is vital that these services are adequately staffed and provided with sufficient resources to enable them to carry out their work.

Appendix: *Check-list for information to be documented during an assessment*

- Level of consciousness
- Psychiatric history and mental state examination
- Social situation and recent life events
- Risk
- Alcohol and drug use
- Decisions taken
- Specific arrangements for follow-up

Source: Royal College of Psychiatrists (1994).

References

BLAKE, D. R. & MITCHELL, J. R. A. (1978) Self-poisoning: management of patients in Nottingham, 1976. *British Medical Journal, i*, 1032–1035.

CATALAN, J., MARSACK, P., HAWTON, K., *et al* (1980) Comparison of doctors and nurses in assessment of deliberate self-poisoning patients. *Psychological Medicine*, 10, 483–491.

COLLIER, J., CUMMINS, T. A. & HAMILTON, M. (1976) A survey of suicidal behaviour in the mid-Essex area in 1972. *Journal of the Royal College of Physicians*, 10, 381–392.

DENNIS, M. S. & LINDESAY, J. (1995) Suicide in the elderly: the United Kingdom perspective. *International Psychogeriatrics*, 7, 263–274.

DEPARTMENT OF HEALTH AND SOCIAL SECURITY (1984) *The Management of Deliberate Self-harm* (HN(84)25). London: Department of Health and Social Security.

ENNIS, J., BARNES, R. A., KENNEDY, S., *et al* (1989) Depression in self-harm patients. *British Journal of Psychiatry*, 154, 41–47.

GARDNER, R., HANKA, R., O'BRIEN, V. C., *et al* (1977) Psychological and social evaluation in cases of deliberate self-poisoning admitted to a general hospital. *British Medical Journal, ii*, 1567–1570.

——, ——, ROBERTS, S. J., *et al* (1982) Psychological and social evaluation in cases of deliberate self-poisoning seen in an accident department. *British Medical Journal*, 284, 491–493.

GIBBONS, J., BUTLER, J., URWIN, P., *et al* (1978) Evaluation of a social work service for self-poisoning patients. *British Journal of Psychiatry*, 133, 111–118.

GILBODY, S., HOUSE, A. & OWENS, D. (1997) Early repetition of deliberate self-harm. *Journal of the Royal College of Physicians of London*, 31, 171–172.

HAMER, D., SANJEEV, D., BUTTERWORTH, E., *et al* (1991) Using the Hospital Anxiety and Depression Scale to screen for psychiatric disorders in people presenting with deliberate self-harm. *British Journal of Psychiatry*, 158, 782–784.

HAWTON, K., BANCROFT, J., CATALAN, J., *et al* (1981) Domiciliary and outpatient treatment of self-poisoning patients by medical and non-medical staff. *Psychological Medicine*, 11, 169–177.

—— & CATALAN, J. (1987) *Attempted Suicide: A Practical Guide to its Nature and Management* (2nd edn). Oxford: Oxford University Press.

——, MCKEOWN, S., DAY, A., *et al* (1987) Evaluation of outpatient counselling compared with general practitioner care following overdoses. *Psychological Medicine*, 17, 751–761.

—— & FAGG, J. (1988) Suicide, and other causes of death, following attempted suicide. *British Journal of Psychiatry*, 152, 359–366.

—— & KIRK, J. W. (1989) Problem solving. In *Cognitive–Behaviour Therapy for Psychiatric Problems: A Practical Guide* (eds K. Hawton, P. Salkovskis, J. W. Kirk & D. Clarke), pp. 406–426. Oxford: Oxford University Press.

—— & JAMES, R. (1995) General hospital services for attempted suicide patients: a survey in one region. *Health Trends*, **27**, 18–21.

——, FAGG, J., SIMKIN, S., *et al* (1997) Trends in deliberate self-harm in Oxford, 1985–1995. Implications for clinical services and the prevention of suicide. *British Journal of Psychiatry*, **171**, 556–560.

——, ARENSMAN, E., TOWNSEND, E., *et al* (1998) Deliberate self harm: systematic review of efficacy of psychosocial and pharmacological treatments in preventing repetition. *British Medical Journal*, **317**, 441–447.

HOUSE, A., OWENS, D. & STORER, D. (1992) Psycho-social intervention following attempted suicide: is there a case for better services? *International Review of Psychiatry*, **4**, 15–22.

—— & HODGSON, G. (1994) Estimating needs and meeting demands. In *Liaison Psychiatry: Defining Needs and Planning Services* (eds S. Benjamin, A. House & P. Jenkins), pp. 3–15. London: Gaskell.

KAPUR, N., HOUSE, A., CREED, F., *et al* (1998) Management of deliberate self-poisoning in adults in teaching hospitals: a descriptive study. *British Medical Journal*, **316**, 831–832.

KENNEDY, P., KREITMAN, N. & OVENSTONE, I. M. K. (1974) The prevalence of suicide and parasuicide ('attempted suicide') in Edinburgh. *British Journal of Psychiatry*, **124**, 36–41.

KREITMAN, N. & FOSTER, J. (1991) Construction and selection of predictive scales, with special reference to parasuicide. *British Journal of Psychiatry*, **159**, 185–192.

LINEHAN, M. M., HEARD, H. L. & ARMSTRONG, H. E. (1993) Naturalistic follow-up of a behavioural treatment for chronically parasuicidal borderline patients. *Archives of General Psychiatry*, **50**, 971–974.

MCLEAVY, B. C., DALY, R. J., LUDGATE, J. W., *et al* (1994) Interpersonal problem-solving skills training in the treatment of self-poisoning patients. *Suicide and Life-Threatening Behaviour*, **24**, 382–394.

MINISTRY OF HEALTH (1961) *Attempted Suicide* (HM(61):94). London: Ministry of Health.

MOLLER, H. J. (1989) Efficacy of different strategies of aftercare for patients who have attempted suicide. *Journal of the Royal Society of Medicine*, **82**, 643–647.

MORGAN, H. G., JONES, E. M. & OWEN, J. H. (1993) Secondary prevention of non-fatal deliberate self-harm. The green card study. *British Journal of Psychiatry*, **163**, 111–112.

NEWSON-SMITH, J. G. B. & HIRSCH, S. R. (1979) A comparison of social workers and psychiatrists in evaluating parasuicide. *British Journal of Psychiatry*, **134**, 335–342.

NORDENTOFT, M., BREUM, L., MUNCK, L. K., *et al* (1993) High mortality by natural and unnatural causes: a 10 year follow-up study of patients admitted to a poisoning treatment centre after suicide attempts. *British Medical Journal*, **306**, 1637–1641.

OWENS, D. (1990) Self-harm patients not admitted to hospital. *Journal of the Royal College of Physicians of London*, **24**, 281–283.

——, DENNIS, M., JONES, S., *et al* (1991) Self-poisoning patients discharged from accident and emergency: risk factors and outcome. *Journal of the Royal College of Physicians of London*, **25**, 218–222.

—— & HOUSE, A. (1994) General hospital services for deliberate self-harm: haphazard clinical provision, little research, no central strategy. *Journal of the Royal College of Physicians of London*, **28**, 370–371.

ROYAL COLLEGE OF PSYCHIATRISTS (1994) *The General Hospital Management of Adult Deliberate Self-Harm: A Consensus Statement on Standards for Service Provision* (CR32). London: Royal College of Psychiatrists.

SAKINOFSKY, I. & ROBERTS, R. S. (1990) Why parasuicides repeat despite problem resolution. *British Journal of Psychiatry*, **156**, 399–405.

SALKOVSKIS, P., ATHA, C. & STORER, D. (1990) Cognitive–behavioural problem solving in the treatment of patients who repeatedly attempt suicide: a controlled study. *British Journal of Psychiatry*, **157**, 871–876.

WATERHOUSE, J. & PLATT, S. (1990) General hospital admission in the management of parasuicide. A randomised controlled trial. *British Journal of Psychiatry*, **156**, 236–242.

WILLIAMS, R. & MORGAN, H. G. (1994) *Suicide Prevention: The Challenge Confronted. A Manual of Guidance for Purchasers and Providers of Mental Health Care.* London: HMSO.

4 Managing behavioural disturbance in the general hospital: facilities and training

ELSPETH GUTHRIE
and ELEANOR FELDMAN

This chapter considers the facilities and training needed in general hospitals for the safe and appropriate management of patients with behavioural disturbance. As David Storer discusses some of these issues in relation to accident and emergency (A&E) departments in Chapter 2, this chapter concentrates more on the needs of in-patient areas. We do, however, give advice on the writing of protocols for use with respect to the observation of disturbed patients, something which most often occurs in the A&E department, and on the particular training needs of A&E staff.

Facilities

Acute psychological disturbance is common in the general medical setting. Each hospital should have a policy regarding the management of acutely disturbed patients. An example of such a policy is given in Appendix 1. Hospitals should develop either a specific area (or areas) or facilities on each ward where patients who are acutely disturbed can be managed. These would be in addition to those available in the A&E department (Chapter 2).

Acutely disturbed patients are best managed in a single-bed room, which needs to be well lit and sparsely furnished. It should be fitted with an appropriate alarm system. The door should have an observational glass panel. If the room is not on the ground floor, the window should be made safe, by fitting reinforced glass and by preventing the window from being fully opened.

Observational policy

Each hospital, and in particular each A&E department, should have written protocols concerning the management of acutely disturbed patients. There should be a written protocol (or observational policy) that clearly indicates the kind of patients, and their degree of disturbance, for which the special observation room should be used. The protocol should also specify the minimum nursing requirements for such patients and the frequency of observation required. The room should never be used for seclusion and a patient should never be left in the room unattended, with the door closed.

Whenever the room is used for a disturbed patient, the level of nursing required should be discussed and agreed between the medical and senior nursing staff on duty. The level of nursing observation required may change during the patient's stay if he or she has recently presented and is being held in an A&E department, and this should be reviewed hourly by the medical and senior nursing staff. No patient should ever be placed in such a room without the above being formally agreed.

The level of observation should be discussed and agreed between senior nursing staff and medical staff and recorded in the patient's medical notes. The notes should specify how closely the patient needs to be observed and how frequently the level of observation needs to be reviewed. If the patient is very disturbed, additional nursing may be required.

A plan should be recorded in the medical case notes that summarises the observational policy and specifies how closely the patient needs to be observed. This plan should be updated whenever the patient is formally reviewed (at least hourly).

Each department should be encouraged to develop individual protocols that reflect local facilities. An example of a written protocol in relation to the use of the special observation room is given in Appendix 2.

Training

Each hospital should have a policy regarding the training of staff in the management of acute psychiatric disturbance (see Appendix 1). One senior member of staff (either medical or nursing) should take a lead in the development of staff training. The policy should clearly stipulate the degree and frequency of training required for each type of staff member. Members of staff working in units where acute disturbance is common, particularly the A&E department, will require more intensive training than members of staff who work in units that rarely deal with acute disturbance.

Training for A&E staff

One member of the senior clinical staff should take the lead in organising and being responsible for training all staff within the department. This would involve the organisation of regular training sessions and the monitoring of individual staff member's requirements for safety training. The training coordinator should receive additional training by attending recognised courses on the management of potentially violent patients.

All staff working in the A&E department should receive regular training on the management of acute psychiatric disturbance. In large departments this could be organised by means of a cascade system.

Junior medical staff who rotate through the department every six months should receive training in communication skills, rapid appraisal of disturbed patients, the pharmacological management of disturbed patients, breakaway techniques and the medico-legal issues. This training must be undertaken within the first two weeks of their appointment.

Senior medical staff, resident in the department, in addition to the above, should receive training in control and restraint techniques.

Nursing staff working in the department should receive training in communication skills, risk assessment triage, breakaway techniques, control and restraint techniques and the medico-legal issues.

Every member of staff should have one half-day every six months devoted to safety training.

The importance of basic communication skills should be emphasised. Many acute episodes of disturbance can be prevented or minimised by the subtle and non-provocative intervention of hospital staff.

Training for staff elsewhere in the hospital

Medical staff who are exposed to potential risk should receive training in the management of the acutely disturbed patient. This should occur on a regular basis and particularly during induction weeks. A written protocol should be developed, which should be available on every ward, outlining the main management strategies for the treatment of the disturbed patients.

All nurses on general wards should be trained in the management of acutely disturbed patients and should be able to produce a nursing care plan that assesses the acute status of the patient and recognises that the patient's mental state may fluctuate. The care plan should be updated every shift. Training should inform nurses of the most common causes of acute disturbance and reinforce the important role of a consistent nursing approach. The degree of training for each nurse should reflect the frequency of contact with acutely disturbed patients. Hospitals with centralised admission wards and centralised facilities for the management of acutely disturbed patients should train staff working in those areas to the same extent as for A&E staff.

General issues

Security staff

In certain circumstances, security staff may be called to help manage a patient who is acutely disturbed and endangering staff. Security staff who are asked to do this must have received training in control and restraint. Security staff must not be used to nurse patients or supplement staff shortages.

Handbooks for junior medical staff

Many trusts now prepare and make available handbooks for junior medical staff. Such a handbook should contain advice and guidance on the assessment and management of all medical emergencies, including acute behavioural disturbance and psychiatric emergencies.

Staff safety

In addition to training in the management of acute disturbance, staff should also be trained in general issues relating to safety. This should include advice about personal responsibility, prevention and break-away techniques. In the event of a violent incident, appropriate reporting and review of the event should take place. Support services and private individual counselling should be available to staff.

Managerial arrangements

In the event of a patient being detained in the general hospital under the Mental Health Act, an arrangement for the managers of the hospital (if a separate National Health Service trust from psychiatry) needs to be made so that they can hold the necessary papers. Their links with relevant officers in the psychiatric services need to be made clear. If the general hospital is a separate trust from the psychiatric hospital trust, there needs to be either a designated person within the general hospital who is properly trained in the administration of the Mental Health Act, or a written agreement whereby clinical staff of the general hospital trust will have access to the relevant Mental Health Act administrator in the psychiatric hospital trust. For further guidance on the use of the Mental Health Act in the general hospital, see Chapter 6.

Appendix 1: Example policy for the management of acute behavioural disturbance in the general hospital

The coordination of services for the management of acutely disturbed patients in the general hospital will be undertaken by a special group of relevant health professionals. The group will be led by Dr X and will include the following: a consultant physician, a consultant psychiatrist, a consultant in A&E medicine, a senior nursing officer, a ward sister, an A&E nurse and a psychiatric nurse.

(1) Definition of acute disturbance

(a) Patients who are at high or moderate risk of self-harm and are making active threats to injure themselves.
(b) Patients who are of high or moderate risk of harm to others.
(c) Other disturbed behaviour that means the patient cannot be safely nursed in bed (e.g. patients who are confused and disoriented, who wander about the ward, who are responding to hallucinations, whose behaviour is unpredictable and disruptive, who are intoxicated or withdrawing from drugs, or who are agitated and difficult to manage).

(2) Facilities

Designated areas within the hospital, wards X and Y, have been specially equipped for the management of patients who are acutely disturbed. Each ward contains four single-bed rooms, which have been specially designed. Each room:

(a) is well lit;
(b) is sparsely furnished with furniture which is bolted to the floor and does not have sharp edges;
(c) is fitted with an appropriate alarm system;
(d) has a door that opens both ways and is fitted with an observational glass panel;
(e) has a reinforced-glass window that opens only partially.

(3) Level of observation

All patients who are acutely disturbed should be observed on a regular basis. An agreed plan of observation and management should be detailed in the medical and nursing notes. Patients should be regularly monitored at least every 15 minutes. If more frequent monitoring than this is required, it should be clearly specified in the medical notes. An observation chart should be kept. The level of observation a patient requires should be reviewed at least every 12 hours.

(4) Training

Nursing staff working on wards X and Y will need a high degree of training in the assessment and management of acute disturbance, communication skills, breakaway techniques and control and restraint techniques. Each nurse should have one half-day every six months devoted to safety training.

Nurses working on other in-patient units should receive training in the assessment and management of acute disturbance and breakaway techniques. Each nurse should have one hour every six months devoted to safety training. As there have been no incidents of acute disturbance in the out-patient setting, nurses working exclusively in the out-patient setting will not require any additional training.

Junior medical staff who rotate through departments every six months should receive training in communication skills, rapid appraisal of disturbed patients, the pharmacological management of disturbed patients and breakaway techniques. This training must be undertaken within the first two weeks of their appointment.

(5) Availability of psychiatric staff

Specialist advice from on-call psychiatrists will be available at all times. The duty psychiatrist should be able to attend within 30 minutes of being called.

(6) Critical incident review

The number of patients with acute disturbance and the treatment and management of such patients should be carefully recorded and audited every six months. This will inform the need for additional training or facilities.

(7) Staff support

Staff involved in violent incidents or the victims of assault should have access to appropriate counselling. This will be arranged through the occupational health department.

(8) Debriefing following major incidents

A debriefing and review session will be arranged for staff involved in any serious major incident. Such an incident will be defined as any that involves physical injury or the threat of severe physical injury to a member of staff, or severe self-injury or suicide of a patient. The meeting will be arranged as soon as possible after the incident and will be attended by all staff involved. The aim of the meeting will be to gather information concerning the incident, review current hospital policy and provide support to staff.

Appendix 2: Example observational policy (protocol regarding the use of the special observation room)

(1) Suitability of patients

   (a) High or moderate risk of self-harm.
   (b) High or moderate risk of harm to others.
   (c) Other disturbed behaviour that cannot be contained elsewhere and that potentially places either the patient or others at risk.

(2) Minimising the risk of self-harm

   (a) Remove articles that could be used to self-harm or injure others.
   (b) If articles (including some articles of clothing) cannot be removed, the patient should be considered to be at high risk.

(3) Level of observation

   (a) All patients placed in the room must be regularly observed.
   (b) The level of observation should be agreed and documented by senior nursing and medical staff.
   (c) As the mental state of the patient may change, the level of observation required should be reviewed every hour.

(4) Frequency of observation

    (a) Constant supervision is required for patients at high risk of active self-harm or harm to others.

    (b) Observation every five minutes is required for patients not actively threatening suicide but at high risk.

    (c) Observation every 15 minutes is required for patients not actively threatening suicide but at moderate risk.

    (d) An observation chart should be used to record each observation.

(5) Use of the observation room should be recorded

The use of the room should be recorded and the kind of patient cared for in the room should be described. This should be audited every six months as part of the department's risk management strategy.

5 Medical management of acute behavioural disturbance in the general hospital

TREVOR FRIEDMAN

There are three common types of patient encountered in the general hospital setting who will need medication for their disturbed behaviour: those with acute confusional states due to underlying organic illness, those with psychiatric illnesses and those with alcohol or drug intoxication.

Assessment

Early intervention and recognition of signs of disturbance are important and a brief assessment of a patient's mental state should be made in the notes on admission to hospital; with elderly patients a more detailed assessment of cognitive function is required.

In cases of disturbed behaviour the patient should be fully assessed, in an environment that will help calm the patient (see below). All information should be carefully recorded: the case notes will provide the best information relating to the patient's state of mind because following medication these symptoms are unlikely to be evident. There should be the expectation that all medical staff can undertake a competent assessment of mental state and record it in clear, professional terminology.

Medication should be used only as part of the overall treatment plan. Discussion should occur between nurses and medical staff as to whether medication is necessary or whether other nursing management should be tried first.

There should be an assessment of the level of disturbance. At the lowest level, patients may be restless or over-aroused but without causing serious concern. Management would be aimed at identification of the cause and preventative interventions. At increased levels of disturbance, patients will be behaving in a disruptive manner that may be preventing them receiving their treatment or interfering with other patients and staff. At the most severe level of disturbance, the behaviour is aggressive or is affecting the patient's treatment to the extent that it is becoming dangerous to health. These patients are more likely to require rapid tranquillisation. The level of disturbance needs to be considered when deciding upon the type and dose of drug (see below).

An assessment will help to differentiate between the various causes of the disturbed mental state. A history from the patient's relatives is often essential and a range of investigations will often be helpful in detecting organic illness. A history of severe mental illness or the presence of delusions, hallucinations and other bizarre behaviour in *clear consciousness* could indicate a psychiatric illness; a history of confusion with disorientation in time, place or person, and possible cognitive impairment would suggest an acute or an acute-on-chronic confusional state. A history of alcohol abuse or abnormal liver function tests is obviously important in identifying an alcohol problem.

General principles

(a) Early intervention is desirable, as disturbed behaviour should be brought under control as soon as possible.
(b) Medication should be used as safely as possible:
  (i)   oral medication is preferable to parenteral administration;
  (ii) dose titration with repeated smaller doses is preferable to large initial doses in cases where the cause of the disturbance is unknown;
  (iii) the patient's mental state and the time and dose of drugs should be carefully recorded;
  (iv) patients should be observed carefully following rapid tranquillisation.
(c) A treatment plan for continuation medication should be recorded and reviewed regularly.

Drug management of acute disturbance

Psychiatric illness

For people suffering from a psychotic illness, a psychiatrist should be contacted as soon as possible. If patients are extremely disturbed and represent a risk to themselves or others, the recommended drug is haloperidol, 5–10 mg orally or intramuscularly. The dose required may be significantly more or less than this on occasion and will depend on factors such as the size and age of the patient, the degree of disturbance and the underlying psychiatric condition. Further doses can be given hourly. In extreme disturbance, lorazepam, 2–4 mg orally or intramuscularly, can be added. If given intramuscularly, lorazepam should be diluted with equal volumes of water. The benzodiazepine antagonist flumazenil should be available in case of respiratory depression.

With known psychiatric patients, evidence from previous notes may suggest that higher doses may be required. The elderly should be treated with half the normal adult doses. There is a possibility of acute dystonic reactions to major tranquillisers; these will respond to procyclidine, 5 mg intramuscularly or orally.

Acute confusional states

Management of these conditions includes the identification and treatment of underlying causes, if possible. If medication is required, small doses of haloperidol should be used, up to 5 mg orally or intramuscularly in the non-elderly and 1 mg orally intramuscularly in the elderly. Patients should be reviewed in an hour. There should be close observation to detect extrapyramidal side-effects.

Alcohol and drug states

If patients in alcohol withdrawal show disturbed behaviour they should be treated acutely with diazepam, 10 mg orally, or dorazepam, 2 mg intramuscularly. Thiamine will help to prevent the complications of alcohol withdrawal. Patients should then be placed on an alcohol-withdrawal regimen.

Patients who are suffering from acute drug or alcohol intoxication or drug withdrawal should be treated with haloperidol, 5 mg orally or intramuscularly. Continuing disturbance should be treated as for 'psychiatric illness'.

After-care

Patients should not be left unattended in the hour after tranquillisation. The level of observation will need to be considered by the medical and nursing team. In the case of the rapid tranquillisation of very disturbed individuals, observations should be made every 15 minutes for one hour and these should be recorded on a form. This observation procedure should include the following.

(a) The level of consciousness should be assessed:
  (i) awake and active;
  (ii) awake and calm;
  (iii) asleep but rousable;
  (iv) asleep and unrousable.

A protocol should be agreed on the appropriate management in situations in which there is an alteration in the level of consciousness.

(b) For levels (iii) or (iv), respiratory rate and past blood pressure and oxygen saturation should be recorded. Arterial gases should be analysed if oxygen saturation is less than 90%.

(c) Blood pressure should be monitored, if possible, if antipsychotic drugs have been given.

(d) There should be reassessment after an hour to look for evidence of dystonia. Basic neurological observation should be carried out. There should be decisions as to whether parenteral or oral medication should be used to keep the situation under control and about the need for specialist advice. There should be further consideration of the treatment plan and levels of nursing and medical observations. There should be a daily reassessment of mental state and specialist advice should be sought if the patient remains disturbed after three days.

Recommended drugs

Table 5.1 lists the drugs recommended for managing these situations (detailed under separate headings below) and Table 5.2 shows the maximum recommended doses. For relatively recent reviews of the use of drugs for rapid tranquillisation see Dubin *et al* (1986), Dubin (1988), Sheard (1988), Ellison *et al* (1989), Goldberg *et al* (1989) and *Drugs and Therapeutics Bulletin* (1991). The American Psychiatric Association (1999) has also produced guidelines on the management of delirium.

Drug interactions

The *British National Formulary* contains further information on drug interactions and this should be consulted for patients taking other drugs including alcohol, antiepileptic drugs, levodopa and lithium.

TABLE 5.1
Recommended drugs for acute behavioural disturbance

Drug	Route of administration
Haloperidol	Intramuscularly or orally
Droperidol	Intramuscularly or orally
Lorazepam	Intramuscularly or orally
Diazepam	Orally
Procyclidine	Intramuscularly, intravenously or orally
Flumazenil	Intravenously
Thiamine	Intramuscularly or orally

TABLE 5.2
Advisory maximum drug doses for the management of acute behavioural disturbance

Drug	Maximum daily dose (mg)	
	Oral	*Intramuscular*
Antipsychotics		
Chlorpromazine	1000	200
Haloperidol	100	60
in extreme situations	200	120?[1]
Droperidol	120	60–90
Methotrimeprazine	1000	200
Benzodiazepines (for anxiety)		
Diazepam	30	60?[1] (120[2])
Lorazepam	4	8?[1]

1. Unclear recommendation – extrapolated from information given.
2. Data sheet for delirium tremens.
Source: British Medical Association & Royal Pharmaceutical Society of Great Britain (1996) and drug manufacturers' data sheets.

Special consideration may be necessary in the use of drugs in medical conditions such as renal failure, heart disease, epilepsy and pregnancy.

Antipsychotics

These have been consistently demonstrated to be safe and effective for rapid tranquillisation (Dubin *et al*, 1986). Hypotension is the most common potentially serious side-effect and appears more often with the less potent drugs, such as chlorpromazine and methotrimeprazine (Dubin *et al*, 1986; Goldberg *et al*, 1989). Sedation and extrapyramidal side-effects are also relatively frequent. The overall rate of side-effects appears to be less than 10% (range 0–33%) in the initial stages but some degree of sedation and extrapyramidal effects occur in most patients over the next few days (Dubin, 1988). The most dangerous complication is cardiorespiratory arrest, the incidence of which is not known.

Parenteral drugs avoid first-pass metabolism and therefore have greater bio-availability, which varies between individuals and drugs (Lader & Herrington, 1990). A reasonable general assumption is about a 2:1 oral:parenteral equivalent dose.

Haloperidol

(a) It is a butyrophenone with minimal cardiorespiratory depressant effects and has been widely studied.

(b) Intramuscular injection brings quicker improvement than oral administration but there appears to be no advantage after three hours (Moller *et al*, 1982).

(c) Significant improvement may occur within 30 minutes of intramuscular injection but in most studies one to two hours is more realistic (Dubin *et al*, 1986).

(d) There are no comparative studies of intramuscular and intravenous haloperidol. In medical patients intravenous haloperidol caused significant improvement within 10–30 minutes (Dudley *et al*, 1979).

(e) Most studies report intramuscular doses of around 5–10 mg repeated every 30–60 minutes (average doses over 24 hours about 40 mg) (Dubin *et al*, 1986).

(f) Single intravenous doses as high as 75 mg, with 240 mg administered over 24 hours, have been reported without serious sequelae in medically ill patients (Adams, 1988).

Droperidol

(a) It is related to haloperidol but is substantially more sedative and transient hypotension appears to be more frequent (Granacher & Ruth, 1979; Adams, 1988). It has a short half-life, which may be practically important if the drug is given parenterally, as the effect may wear off quickly.

(b) It is very rapidly absorbed after intramuscular administration (peak plasma concentration is reached within 20 minutes), so there is doubtful advantage in giving it intravenously (Cressman *et al*, 1973).

(c) A comparison of droperidol and haloperidol in 27 acutely agitated patients found that 64% and 19%, respectively, responded within 30 minutes (Resnick & Burton, 1984). It has been queried whether it is clinically less effective than haloperidol (Adams, 1988).

(d) Intramuscular doses in studies have been around 5–12.5 mg every 15–30 minutes, as necessary (Granacher & Ruth, 1979; Resnick & Burton, 1984).

Chlorpromazine

(a) It is a low-potency sedative.

(b) A comparison of intramuscular chlorpromazine and haloperidol in 30 acutely disturbed patients showed equal tranquillisation, but two of the 15 on chlorpromazine collapsed with severe hypotension (Man & Chen, 1973).

Benzodiazepines

These are sedative drugs of low toxicity. The principal adverse effect is respiratory depression. Flumazenil allows rapid reversal of respiratory depression (but its half-life of one hour means repeated administration may be necessary) (Whitwam, 1988). Further concerns are about paradoxical disinhibition and dependence. Paradoxical disinhibition or feelings of increased hostility are reported to have an incidence of under 1%, equal to that of placebo in controlled studies of benzodiazepines. Overt behavioural disturbance is even less frequent (Dietch & Jennings, 1988). Nearly all cases of paradoxical disinhibition have been in the context of repeated dosage.

Diazepam

(a) It is poorly and erratically absorbed after intramuscular injection (Greenblatt & Koch-Weser, 1976).

(b) Accumulation is likely with repeated doses (Mandelli *et al*, 1978).

(c) Intravenous diazepam is effective in calming behavioural disturbance within 15 minutes (Pilowsky *et al*, 1992).

(d) Intravenous diazepam causes less venous inflammation than lorazepam.

Lorazepam

(a) In a small study in manic patients the timing of the peak reduction in agitation was: 60–120 minutes when given orally; 45–75 minutes when given intramuscularly; and 5–10 minutes when given intravenously (Modell *et al*, 1985).

(b) In general, intramuscular lorazepam appears as effective as intramuscular haloperidol and has fewer adverse effects (Dubin, 1988).

(c) Its possible advantages over haloperidol have been described. It appears to be more effective than haloperidol in the first two hours with patients already receiving antipsychotic drugs (Salzman *et al*, 1991); 10 patients who received lorazepam on one occasion and haloperidol on another spent less time in seclusion after lorazepam (Bick & Hannah, 1986).

(d) Doses in studies have been 2–10 mg every one to two hours. The maximum single dose reported was 40 mg and maximum daily doses have been around 20–40 mg (Deberdt, 1975; Modell *et al*, 1985; Lenox *et al*, 1986). There are no reports of serious adverse effects with its use over one to two weeks, although ataxia has occurred at doses above 10 mg a day, as have nausea and confusion at the highest doses.

(e) When given by intramuscular injection it should be diluted with an equal volume of sterile water or saline.

Combination treatment with an antipsychotic and benzodiazepine

(a) The most studied combination has been parenteral haloperidol with lorazepam; it is claimed that this reduces the total dose of antipsychotic required (Greenblatt & Raskin, 1986).

(b) There is no clear evidence of increased risk of cardiorespiratory depression and the combination has been given intravenously to severely medically ill patients (Adams, 1988). There are, however, case reports where the intravenous combination has caused cardiorespiratory arrest (Pilowsky *et al*, 1992; Quenstedt *et al*, 1992).

(c) In an open trial the combination given intramuscularly was effective more rapidly (within 30 minutes) than either drug alone (nearer 60 minutes) in most patients (Garza-Trevino *et al*, 1989).

Acknowledgement

I would like to thank Dr Ian Anderson, Senior Lecturer in Manchester, for his advice on the pharmacological aspects of management.

References

ADAMS, F. (1988) Emergency intravenous sedation of the delirious, medically ill patient. *Journal of Clinical Psychiatry*, **49**, 22–27.

AMERICAN PSYCHIATRIC ASSOCIATION (1999) *Practice Guidelines for the Treatment of Patients with Delirium.* Washington, DC: American Psychiatric Association.

BICK, P. A. & HANNAH, A. L. (1986) Intramuscular lorazepam to restrain violent patients. *Lancet, i,* 206.

BRITISH MEDICAL ASSOCIATION & ROYAL PHARMACEUTICAL SOCIETY OF GREAT BRITAIN (1996) *British National Formulary* (March, number 31). London: BMA & Pharmaceutical Press.

CRESSMAN, W. A., PLOSTNIEKS, J. & JOHNSON, P. C. (1973) Absorption, metabolism and excretion of droperidol by human subjects following intramuscular and intravenous administration. *Anesthesiology*, **38**, 363–369.

DEBERDT, R. (1975). Treatment of acute anxiety and agitation by intravenous administration of lorazepam. *Current Medical Research and Opinion*, **3**, 459–463.

DIETCH, J. T. & JENNINGS, R. K. (1988) Aggressive dyscontrol in patients treated with benzodiazepines. *Journal of Clinical Psychiatry*, **49**, 184–187.

DRUGS AND THERAPEUTICS BULLETIN (1991) Management of behavioural emergencies. *Drugs and Therapeutics Bulletin*, **29**, 62–64.

DUBIN, W. R. (1988) Rapid tranquilization: antipsychotics or benzodiazepines? *Journal of Clinical Psychiatry*, **49**, 5–11.

——, WEISS, K. J. & DORN, J. M. (1986) Pharmacotherapy of psychiatric emergencies. *Journal of Clinical Psychopharmacology*, **6**, 210–222.

DUDLEY, D. L., ROWLETT, D. B. & LOEBEL, P. J. (1979) Emergency use of intravenous haloperidol. *General Hospital Psychiatry*, **1**, 240–246.

ELLISON, J., HUGHES, D. & KIMBERLEY, A. W. (1989) An emergency psychiatry update. *Hospital and Community Psychiatry*, **40**, 250–260.

GARZA-TREVINO, E. S., HOLLISTER, L. E., OVERALL, J. E., *et al* (1989) Efficacy of combinations of intramuscular antipsychotics and sedative-hypnotics for control of psychotic agitation. *American Journal of Psychiatry*, **146**, 1598–1601.

GOLDBERG, R. J., DUBIN, W. R. & FOGEL, B. S. (1989) Behavioural emergencies. *Clinical Neuropharmacology*, **12**, 233–248.

GRANACHER, R. P. & RUTH, D. D. (1979) Droperidol in acute agitation. *Current Therapeutic Research*, **25**, 361–365.

GREENBLATT, D. J. & KOCH-WESER, J. (1976) Intramuscular injection of drugs. *New England Journal of Medicine*, **295**, 542–546.

—— & RASKIN, A. (1986) Benzodiazepines: new indications. *Psychopharmacology Bulletin*, **22**, 77–78.

LADER, M. & HERRINGTON, R. (1990) *Biological Treatments in Psychiatry.* Oxford: Oxford University Press.

LENOX, R. H., MODELL, J. G. & WEINER, S. (1986) Acute treatment of manic agitation with lorazepam. *Psychosomatics*, **27**, 28–31.

MAN, P. L. & CHEN, C. H. (1973) Rapid tranquilization of acutely psychotic patients with intramuscular haloperidol and chlorpromazine. *Psychosomatics*, **14**, 59–63.

MANDELLI, M., TOGNONI, G. & GARATTINI, S. (1978) Clinical pharmacokinetics of diazepam. *Clinical Pharmacokinetics*, **3**, 72–91.

MODELL, J. G., LENOX, R. H. & WEINER, S. (1985) Inpatient clinical trial of lorazepam for the management of manic agitation. *Journal of Clinical Psychopharmacology*, **5**, 109–113.

MOLLER, H. J., KISSLING, W. & LANG, C. (1982) Efficacy and side effects of haloperidol in psychotic patients: oral versus intravenous administration. *American Journal of Psychiatry*, **139**, 1571–1575.

PILOWSKY, L. S., RING, H., SHINE, P. J., *et al* (1992) Rapid tranquillisation: a survey of emergency prescribing in a general psychiatric hospital. *British Journal of Psychiatry*, **160**, 831–835.

QUENSTEDT, M., RAMSAY, R. & BERNANDT, M. (1992) Rapid tranquillisation. *British Journal of Psychiatry*, **161**, 573.

RESNICK, M. & BURTON, B. T. (1984) Droperidol vs haloperidol in the initial management of acutely agitated patients. *Journal of Clinical Psychiatry*, **45**, 298–299.

SALZMAN, C., SOLOMON, D., MIYAWAKI, E., *et al* (1991) Parenteral lorazepam versus parenteral haloperidol for the control of psychotic disruptive behavior. *Journal of Clinical Psychiatry*, **52**, 177–180.

SHEARD, M. H. (1988) Review: clinical pharmacology of aggressive behaviour. *Clinical Neuropharmacology*, **11**, 483–492.

WHITWAM, J. G. (1988) Flumazenil: a benzodiazepine antagonist. *British Medical Journal*, **297**, 999–1000.

6 Use of the Mental Health Act and common law in the general hospital

ELEANOR FELDMAN

This chapter covers the application of the Mental Health Act 1983 and common law principles in England and Wales with respect to the management of behaviourally disturbed patients in National Health Service general hospitals. Much of the contents of this chapter are the result of discussions with colleagues and Mental Health Act Commissioners that took place at a conference at Stamford in Lincolnshire in December 1995 (see Acknowledgements).

The Mental Health Act 1983

Unlike other aspects of clinical care, medico-legal issues do not necessarily cross national boundaries. In the UK alone, there are three Mental Health Acts (MHAs) currently in force, one for Scotland (1984), one for Northern Ireland (1986) and one for England and Wales (1983). The Republic of Ireland also has its own Act (1945). My own clinical experience has been in England and the discussions I have had with colleagues and MHA Commissioners have mainly focused on the 1983 Act. There is a need for similar guidance in each jurisdiction. For comment on the law in Scotland, see Carson *et al* (1999).

The use of the MHA is clear with respect to individuals who are suffering from those psychiatric illnesses generally agreed by psychiatrists to fall within its remit. These include functional psychoses such as schizophrenia and affective psychoses. This clarity results from many years of established practice, including tribunals involving lay members and lawyers, the Act's use by staff who have been appropriately trained and who are familiar with its workings, and the monitoring and advice of the MHA Commission. However, there is far less experience and agreement regarding the inclusion within the MHA of diagnostic categories that can be interpreted flexibly under the current wording of the Act, for example delirium or neurotic conditions compromising medical care, and uncertainty exists in settings where medical and nursing staff caring for the patients are unfamiliar with the principles and practice of the MHA.

The MHA does not generally apply to the detention and treatment of patients for physical illness, for which they must give informed consent, or be treated under common law. However, what is the position where the physical illness itself results in disability of mind through disordered brain function, or where the effects of self-harm need treatment and are the consequence of disturbed behaviour in a mentally disordered person? Was it intended that the MHA be used in these situations? If it was, then logically all non-psychiatric medical and surgical and nursing staff should be trained in its use. As it is, they are not, but turn to liaison psychiatrists for assistance.

The remit of the Act

The MHA allows for the legal detention and treatment of persons with mental illness, mental impairment and psychopathic disorder where admission is considered necessary in the interest of their health or safety, or for the protection of others, and where they are unable or unwilling to consent to such admission. It is an enabling Act and does not have to be used in all instances of the above, but its use will provide certain legal safeguards for patients and for staff responsible for the patients subject to the MHA.

While any mental disorder can fall within the remit of the MHA, in practice there are common circumstances where restraint and treatment are applied without recourse to the Act. In these situations, the actions performed (if carried out without the real consent of the patient) can be defended only if they are within the scope of the common law.

In section 1 of the MHA, mental disorder is defined broadly. Section 1(2) states: "'mental disorder' means mental illness, arrested or incomplete development of mind, psychopathic disorder and any other disorder or disability of mind and 'mentally disordered' shall be construed accordingly", and this includes temporary states of mental disturbance such as delirium and intoxication (subject to exclusion under section 1(3) of the Act – see below), as well as more prolonged conditions such as dementia and brain damage.

It should be noted in particular that someone who is intoxicated with alcohol or drugs and who is judged to have the capacity to refuse essential intervention may in certain circumstances legitimately be subject to the MHA, although there must be grounds for intervention other than alcohol or drug addiction alone: section 1(3) states that the Act cannot be applied to persons by "reason only of promiscuity or other immoral conduct, sexual deviancy or dependence on alcohol or drugs".

Although not appropriate for the treatment of physical disorder *per se*, the MHA may apply where physical disorder contributes to mental disorder or is otherwise inextricably linked with the mental disorder (see *Re K.B.* [1993] 19 BMLR 144; *B. v. Croydon Health Authority* [1995] 1 All ER 683), such as feeding in anorexia nervosa and the use of thyroxine in mental disorder caused by hypothyroidism. It does not apply in situations where the treatment of the physical illness will not affect the mental disturbance; this area falls within the scope of the common law (*Re C (Adult: Refusal of Treatment)* [1994] 1 WLR 290) (but see Postscript).

The use of holding orders

Sections 5(2) and 5(4), which relate to the emergency medical and nursing holding orders for those who are already voluntary in-patients, are not applicable in accident and emergency departments, which are regarded as an out-patient setting. Patients cannot be conveyed to another hospital under section 5(2) or 5(4). Where different National Health Service hospital trusts operate on the same site, it is advisable for the respective trust managers formally to agree to act on each other's behalf with respect to the MHA.

Any consultant in charge of a patient's care is the responsible medical officer (RMO) with respect to the MHA; therefore, according to the law, consultant physicians and surgeons may detain their own in-patients using section 5(2). In general hospitals, the initials RMO are frequently applied to the resident medical officer, who is usually only of senior house officer grade; it is therefore very important to be clear that, where the term RMO is applied in respect of the MHA, it always refers to the consultant with medical responsibility for the case.

The MHA allows for the nomination of a deputy by any RMO and this deputy must be a registered medical practitioner (*not* a pre-registration house officer). Consultant physicians and surgeons may therefore nominate their own juniors, of senior house officer grade or above, to act as their deputy. Whether or not this is a good practice is another matter. The *Code of Practice* on the use of the MHA

(Department of Health & Welsh Office, 1999) has advised that only consultant psychiatrists should nominate a deputy and that where RMOs of another speciality wish to detain their own patient, they should make immediate contact with a psychiatrist. Problems can arise if junior physicians are left to invoke the powers of section 5(2) because they and their seniors are often unclear about the precise nature and scope of the powers, the powers may not be administered correctly and the patient may not be assessed by an approved psychiatrist with a view to an admission order or termination of the holding order. An audit carried out at Leeds demonstrated various failings in the use of section 5(2) when it was left to physicians to invoke the power (Buller *et al*, 1996).

The use of the place of safety order and the role of the police

Section 136 empowers the police to detain and take to a place of safety an individual who falls within its remit. It does not relate to emergency admissions. Its purpose is to enable the police to take such persons somewhere where they can safely be assessed by two doctors and an approved social worker with a view to detention under the MHA. There is no official documentation for section 136.

Police may legitimately escort to hospital patients who request their help or those who require hospital treatment but are incapable of consenting. However, they should not bring individuals *against their will* to a hospital unless under section 136 of the MHA and where, by local agreement, the hospital is the designated place of safety. In many districts, hospitals are not the designated place of safety, but the police cells are. The Royal College of Psychiatrists (1997) has commented on the inadvisability of making a hospital a place of safety. Accident and emergency departments, far from being safe places for severely mentally disturbed individuals, are often ill equipped to deal with the kind of people that the police pick up, and hospital staff and other ill patients in the vicinity may be placed at risk.

Managerial arrangements for the MHA

Managers of general hospitals need to make arrangements for the receipt and holding of section papers. The links with relevant officers in the psychiatric hospitals need to be made clear. If the general hospital belongs to a different trust to the psychiatric hospital, there needs to be either a designated person within the general hospital who is properly trained in the administration of the MHA, or a written agreement whereby clinical staff of the general hospital will have access to the relevant MHA officer in the psychiatric trust.

The nature of common law

What is the common law?

The common law refers to that body of rights, duties, obligations and liabilities recognised by the courts over the years. It is made up of principles identified by judges, and has adapted and changed to meet the needs of particular cases or particular developments in our society. This 'judge-revealed law' is to be distinguished from statute law, which comprises the rules and regulations agreed by the authority of Parliament. When the common law principles have been identified, their application to changed sets of circumstances (i.e. to modern problems) should follow. Lord Donaldson, former Master of the Rolls, referred to the common law as 'common sense under a wig'.

When does common law apply?

Common law principles may assist where there are no statutory protections or mechanisms in play. In England and Wales, the MHA 1983 is the relevant codifying statute and where its provisions apply there is little room for the common law principles. On issues where the statute law is silent, the lawfulness of any act or omission is tested by the application of the common law.

What common law principles may be applicable to the treatment of mentally disturbed individuals?

Assumption of capacity in adults

The starting point is the recognition in common law that every adult has the right and capacity to decide whether or not to accept medical treatment, even if a refusal may risk permanent damage to his or her physical or mental health, or even lead to premature death. The reasons for the refusal are irrelevant. Capacity is a legal concept and concerns the ability to understand what is being proposed and the consequences of either refusing or accepting the advice given, and to weigh these issues in the balance in reaching a decision. In law, pre-registration house officers are not qualified to assess a patient's capacity to accept or refuse treatment but all registered medical practitioners are (British Medical Association & Law Society, 1995). Where mental disorder is present or likely, psychiatric involvement is necessary for a proper assessment of capacity, for example in a patient who has made a suicide attempt.

Necessity

The courts have recognised the existence of a common law principle of 'necessity' and have extended it to cover situations where action is required to assist another person without his or her consent. Although such a situation will usually be some form of emergency, the power to intervene is not created by that emergency but derived from the principle of necessity. In *Black* v. *Forsey* (House of Lords, *The Times*, 31 May 1988), Lord Griffiths, when dealing with the common law power to restrain a dangerous lunatic, said that the power was:

> "confined to imposing temporary restraint on a lunatic who has run amok and is a manifest danger either to himself or to others – a state of affairs as obvious to a layman as to a doctor. Such a common law power is confined to the short period necessary before the lunatic can be handed over to the proper authority."

In common language, the judge is pointing out that it is appropriate to act to restrain people believed to be suffering from mental disorder and who are exhibiting behaviour that suggests they are a risk to themselves or others, but where they have not yet been detained under the MHA. In practice, there is usually a period of time when patients who are about to be made subject to the MHA will have to be restrained before the formalities of the Act can be completed. It is also quite common for such patients to require some sedation before the completion of these formalities. Such actions will be defensible if carried out as a necessity and using the minimum intervention required.

Actions performed out of necessity should not continue for an unreasonable length of time, but progress should be made either to a situation of consent or to the use of powers under the MHA. It is not possible to define precisely what is a reasonable or unreasonable length of time, as this would vary with the particular circumstances of each case.

Duty of care

Common law imposes a duty of care on all professional staff to all persons within a hospital; by assuming the responsibility of a particular clinical staff appointment, and professing professional expertise, an individual undertakes to provide proper care for those needing it. Staff may be negligent by omission. Actions involving the use of reasonable restraint and driven by professional responsibility in circumstances of necessity are supported by common law.

As well as individual staff, hospitals also have duties, for example to provide backup staff who are properly trained to assist with aggressive, uncooperative patients in a casualty department, and the hospital must ensure that such staff are authorised to act if necessary. Many hospitals experience problems with fulfilling this duty because they fail to train the security staff in this role, and commonly such staff are disinclined to assist in necessary restraint as they believe that they will be exposed to the risk of litigation for assault. This is a key area for improved staff training and the involvement of the hospital's risk management advisers.

The Bolam test

Where clinical decisions are being made, an individual clinician's competence will be judged against what is considered reasonable and proper by a body of responsible doctors at that time, as ascertained in court from expert testimony. This is termed the Bolam test (*Bolam* v. *Friern Hospital Management Committee* [1957] 2 All ER 118–128 at 122).

The law applied to clinical situations

Having covered the principles underlying the relevant law in the jurisdiction of England and Wales, I now consider their practical application in a number of case vignettes. All the cases have been invented for illustrative purposes. The advice given is not intended to be prescriptive, but to provide an illustration of how the principles discussed above may be applied in practice. In the law, as in medicine, there is always a place for considered judgement, according to the particular circumstances of each case.

Acute organic brain syndrome

A 54-year-old man on the high-dependency unit is recovering from a cardiac arrest that required prolonged resuscitation. As he emerges from several days of coma, he becomes acutely distressed, disoriented and paranoid. He requires heparin for his prosthetic heart valves, and anti-arrhythmia drugs, but refuses to have either and is walking about, dressed and demanding to leave. He has already tried to push past you and the nursing staff. You assess that the only way to help him is to restrain and sedate him against his will, keeping him on the high-dependency medical unit.

This man's refusal is not based on any real understanding of his circumstances and, in delirium, he has no grasp of his risk; it is very clearly in his best interests for him to be detained and sedated so that he can have life-saving treatments. Any reasonable lay person would not dispute this man's need for treatment and would consider hospital staff negligent if they knowingly allowed him to leave and failed to do whatever was necessary to help him.

The MHA *could* be applied for detention and sedation to treat the delirium (a form of mental illness), but delirium is not a situation in which the MHA is commonly used. Such patients are more often detained and treated without recourse to the MHA in view of the transient nature of the disturbance, the (so far) undisputed need for intervention and the evident lack of capacity to give meaningful consent or refusal. However, if strong measures are required, such as the use of psychiatric nursing staff to pin this man to his bed while he is forcibly injected with haloperidol, or if the situation persists over a prolonged period, it may be advisable to use the MHA. The order should be cancelled as soon as the patient has recovered mentally.

Treatments other than sedation in this case are not authorised by the MHA, but are justifiably given in a legal sense if the post-registration physician directing the treatment has judged that the patient does not have the capacity to make a meaningful refusal. The same legal decision *could* also apply to the use of sedation, in which case a psychiatrist need not be involved, as, in law, any registered medical practitioner is considered able to judge a patient's capacity to consent (British Medical Association & Law Society, 1995). This does not apply to patients detained under the MHA after the first three months of treatment; only the RMO is then judged to be able to determine a patient's capacity to consent.

Patient refusing medical intervention after deliberate self-harm

A 30-year-old man is brought to the accident and emergency department after taking an overdose of 70 paracetamol tablets four hours earlier. There is no history available and the patient refuses to say anything about himself other than he wants to be left alone to die. He refuses to give blood for a determination of paracetamol concentration and refuses any medical intervention. Can medical treatment be given without his consent?

This illustrates a fairly common scenario. The patient presents the medical staff with the dilemma of whether they should assume he has full capacity to refuse medical treatment, in which case they might leave him to suffer the consequences of liver failure, possibly death, or whether they should act out of necessity and as part of their duty of care to treat someone in whom capacity may reasonably be in doubt and where the patient could be mentally ill. A psychiatrist will not be in a position to assess the patient fully for mental disorder before the harmful effects of paracetamol become irreversible, but should be called to assist in the assessment of capacity. My own position on such cases is to take it that there are usually good grounds for reasonable doubt with respect to the patient's capacity to make a fully informed and reasoned choice and proceed with whatever action is necessary to save his life under the common law. Is it better for a clinician to have a living patient who may sue for assault for saving the life he no longer wants, or to have a dead patient with grieving relatives who may sue for negligence? There are currently no precedents either way.

Intoxicated patient refusing to cooperate with assessment following deliberate self-harm

> A young man is brought to the accident and emergency department by paramedics who found him lying in a doorway with a suicide note and an empty bottle of paracetamol. He is intoxicated with alcohol, belligerent, refuses to talk to any staff and is making moves to leave. You have no other information and have to make a decision as to whether or not to let him go.

This case typifies a common clinical problem faced by accident and emergency staff and psychiatrists covering accident and emergency departments. If there is sufficient concern to warrant detaining this patient for further assessment of a possible underlying mental disorder, then use of the MHA is certainly justified. The fact that the patient is intoxicated is not an obstacle to the use of the MHA, as the Act is not being used to detain or treat someone because of alcohol misuse or dependence alone (see above regarding section 1(3)), but because of the concern that there may be an underlying mental disorder that is temporarily obscured by intoxication and lack of cooperation.

Anorexia nervosa patient *in extremis* and refusing food

> A 19-year-old woman weighing only four stone (25 kg) has been admitted to the acute medical unit. She consents to a saline drip, but not to any dextrose or parenteral feeding. She is close to death from starvation.

The MHA is frequently used in relation to patients with anorexia who are close to death to authorise feeding as part of both the psychiatric and the physical treatment of these patients. Experts in eating disorders regard refeeding as an essential first step in the psychiatric treatment, as starvation itself produces distorted thinking. There are legal precedents to support this view, notably *Re K.B.* (see above). The MHA Commission (1997) has issued a guidance note on this particular topic that discusses the legal issues in more detail.

Anorexia nervosa patient with diabetes, refusing insulin

> The same patient as above now also has insulin-dependent diabetes; this time she agrees to feeding, but refuses insulin, since she knows that she will not gain weight without it. She would die if you agreed to this plan.

I would take the view that there is no difference between this case and the preceding situation. Insulin is as essential for healthy weight gain as is food; hence, its administration would also form part of the psychiatric treatment plan under section 3 of the MHA. There is currently no legal precedent on this precise point.

Patient with schizophrenia refusing surgery, but accepting other medical care

> A 59-year-old man with chronic schizophrenia is a long-stay patient under section 3. He develops a gangrenous foot and the surgeon's advice is to proceed to amputation. The patient refuses surgery on the grounds that he does not want an amputation, but he agrees to antibiotics and all other forms of treatment. The surgeon asks if the operation can be carried out as part of treatment under section 3 and he impresses upon you his conviction that the patient is likely to die without the amputation.

The MHA should not apply here unless the treatment of the physical disorder would improve the patient's mental disorder. Precedent on this (*Re C* – see above) found that a patient's gangrenous leg could not be amputated as the patient's refusal of surgery was unrelated to his chronic schizophrenia (i.e. he had the capacity to refuse and this refusal was not part of his psychotic thinking) and surgery would not improve his mental condition.

As a general rule, where physical illness and mental disorder coexist, and the issue of treatment under the MHA arises, the clinician must establish:

(a) whether or not the refusal is a valid one in a patient with the capacity to make a decision on this issue;
(b) whether treatment of the physical illness would make a difference to the mental disorder.

Where the treatment of physical illness does ameliorate the mental disorder, then it is also the case that this is treatment of the mental disorder (as in the cases with anorexia) and use of the MHA is justified. If refusal of physical treatment is not the result of the mental disorder, and the treatment is unlikely to make any difference to the mental disorder, then use of the MHA would not be justified (as in this case). If refusal is the result of the mental disorder, but treatment would not ameliorate the mental disorder, then whether the MHA can be used to justify the treatment has become a matter of recent controversy (see below), although treatment of the physical illness may be justifiable under common law as the patient's capacity to either consent or refuse may reasonably be in doubt.

Postscript

Since the meeting at Stamford mentioned above, interpretation of the appeal court judge's ruling in the case of *B. v. Croydon Health Authority* has given rise to some controversy, current at the time of writing, in correspondence in the *British Medical Journal* (Hassan *et al*, 1999; Hewson, 1999; Hull *et al*, 1999). The first contribution was written by accident and emergency doctors who produced an algorithm in consultation with lawyers, but did not consult with psychiatrists or the MHA Commission. The authors stated that: "If the overdose is considered to be a consequence of a mental disorder then the patient can also be treated medically for the overdose under the terms of the MHA." It was this sentence and the corresponding box in the algorithm that sparked a large electronic correspondence in the journal Web pages from concerned psychiatrists who considered this would lead to demands for patients to be placed under a section of the MHA purely to treat the physical consequences of an overdose. The appeal court judge's comments in his summing up included: "It would seem to me strange if a hospital could, without the patient's consent give him treatment directed to alleviating a ... disorder showing itself in suicidal tendencies, but not without such consent be able to treat the consequences of a suicide attempt."

Correspondence has clarified that patients would first have to fulfil the usual criteria for applying the MHA, and then justification according to the appeal court judge's ruling in *B. v. Croydon Health Authority* would come into play only if patients lacked capacity to consent or refuse medical treatment for the physical consequences of their self-harm. This would be a decision for the psychiatric consultant who was the RMO under the Act. In these circumstances, it is unlikely that a patient who was appropriately under a section allowing treatment would also have full capacity to make such a grave decision if it was the mental disorder that led to the self-harm in the first place. As the appeal court judge in *B. v. Croydon Health Authority* also found that B lacked capacity, it was not necessary to invoke the Act in her case either, although the court did with respect to enforced feeding in borderline personality disorder.

We must await further case law or new statute law for clarification on what remains a difficult area.

Acknowledgements

I am grateful to the following who participated in discussions on medico-legal issues at the Stamford meeting: Elspeth Guthrie, Trevor Friedman, Robert Peveler, Nigel Pleming QC, Simon Wessely and Anthony Zigmond. I am also grateful to Allan House for his comments on the subject.

References

BRITISH MEDICAL ASSOCIATION & LAW SOCIETY (1995) *Assessment of Mental Capacity: Guidance for Doctors and Lawyers.* London: British Medical Association.

BULLER C., STORER D. & BENNETT R. (1996) A survey of general hospital in-patients detained under Section 5(2) of the 1983 Mental Health Act. *Psychiatric Bulletin,* **20,** 733–735.

CARSON, A. J., CRICHTON, S., BELL, D., *et al* (1999) When medicine meets the law – guidelines for decision making in acute medical admissions. *Health Bulletin,* **57,** 267–276.

DEPARTMENT OF HEALTH & WELSH OFFICE (1999) *Code of Practice Mental Health Act (1983).* London: Stationery Office.

HASSAN, T. B., MACNAMARA, A. F., DAVY, A., *et al* (1999) Managing patients with deliberate self harm who refuse treatment in the accident and emergency department. *British Medical Journal,* **319,** 107–109.

HEWSON, B. (1999) The law on managing patients who deliberately harm themselves and refuse treatment. *British Medical Journal,* **319,** 905–907.

HULL, A., HAUT, F., FELDMAN, E., *et al* (1999) Correspondence. *British Medical Journal,* **319,** 916–919.

MENTAL HEALTH ACT COMMISSION (1997) *Guidance on the Treatment of Anorexia Nervosa under the Mental Health Act 1983* (Guidance Note 3). London: Mental Health Act Commission.

ROYAL COLLEGE OF PSYCHIATRISTS (1997) *Standards of Places of Safety under Section 136 of the Mental Health Act (1983).* Council Report CR61. London: Royal College of Psychiatrists.

7 Trauma

RICHARD MAYOU

Rapid access to specialist psychiatric *consultation* is necessary in accident and emergency departments for the many patients with disturbances of behaviour or evidence of major psychiatric disorder. However, few hospitals have any form of organised psychiatric *liaison* with emergency care (see Chapter 2); even fewer have any special provision for patients who have suffered trauma. It is easy to make out a case of need but difficult to cite examples of the need having been met. This chapter therefore has to describe the nature of the clinical problems associated with trauma and the evidence on the efficacy of intervention, and then propose ways in which psychological and social help may best be provided. The resultant blueprint is not idealistic, but rather an attainable minimum for good care.

Although the chapter concentrates on *hospital-based services*, the importance of psychological care of trauma within *primary care* should not be overlooked. As will be described, minor trauma can have major psychological consequences; general practitioners need to recognise this and be able to provide care themselves as well as having access to specialist services. This means that consultation–liaison expertise should not be limited to hospital emergency attenders, but available to trauma victims wherever they initially consult, at work, in primary care or elsewhere. This chapter is arranged under the following headings:

    (a) general issues;
    (b) general psychological and social consequences of trauma;
    (c) specific aspects of the type of trauma;
    (d) general principles of care;
    (e) special clinical problems;
    (f) service implications;
    (g) conclusions.

General issues

Epidemiology

Trauma, physical and psychological, is extremely common, although only a proportion is reported to doctors. In total, it is responsible for very considerable morbidity and health care costs (Burdett-Smith, 1992; Driscoll, 1992; Evans & Evans, 1992). Severe injury, most usually following road traffic accidents or falls, is among the leading causes of death, especially in children and younger adults, and of major physical disability. Major trauma, requiring intensive specialist care, is estimated to suffered by no more than 1 in 1000 accident department attenders (Burdett-Smith, 1992).

Less severe injuries have a wider range of causes. Apart from the physical consequences, they have a major impact on absence from work or school, limitations of everyday activity and financial status. The costs in human suffering and the economic costs for health services are very large. While hospital trauma services manage the most severe injuries, they are also responsible for the care of many people who have minor or even no physical injury, whose trauma has been principally psychological.

Medical services

In 1990 there were 256 accident and emergency departments in the UK, which were each dealing with more than 20 000 patients a year – more than 10.5 million people in all. In addition, there were 380 smaller units.

Psychological services must be based on an understanding of the principles of physical care. The nature, outcome and specialist medical management of trauma have never attracted as much attention as the size of the problem requires (Burdett-Smith, 1992).

It is only recently that specialist trauma services have been developed. The present service model for acute care comprises three parts:

   (a) Large specialised *centres* for the management of very severe injuries. These require multi-disciplinary medical and nursing teams to provide acute medical and surgical care as well as to initiate specialist continuing treatment. There is continuing uncertainty about the value of designating a number of these centres as having clear, regional responsibilities for the specialist treatment of major trauma.

TABLE 7.1
Types of trauma

Main categories	Subcategories
Deliberate self-harm	
Accidental injury	Road traffic accident injury
	Domestic injury
	Occupational
	Sport and leisure
Non-accidental injury/assault	Non-sexual
	Sexual
Disasters	

(b) A much greater number of *hospital accident and emergency departments*, offering trauma care. These acute trauma services need to have close working relationships with other specialist services, including those for the care of severe head injury, plastic surgery, burns units and spinal injury units.

(c) Simpler care in health centres, places of work and other settings.

Although hospital-based trauma care is increasingly seen as multi-disciplinary, the focus in practice and in planning is overwhelmingly concerned with physical problems. Awareness of the social and psychological impact has not resulted in any adequate guidelines for the provision of psychosocial care. There has been particular neglect of the longer-term consequences, whether or not they are associated with continuing physical problems.

Only a minority of attenders receive continuing out-patient follow-up care. This means that the opportunities for any form of psychological intervention within the emergency department may be limited, and that later recognition and provision of treatment must involve coordination with primary care and other social, voluntary and community services.

Types of trauma

Each type of trauma (Table 7.1) and its specialist treatment have particular meaning and implications for patients and families, and the liaison psychiatrist will need to be aware of these in assessment, planning individual treatment and organising treatment services.

Relatives, staff and others who may be involved

In addition, we need to be aware of the needs of others who may need psychological help after a trauma:

(a) non-injured participants and bystanders;
(b) relatives;
(c) staff of the emergency department;
(d) others involved in coping with trauma – paramedical and voluntary services, police and so on.

Some relatives accompany victims to the emergency department, while others are summoned urgently and probably many more have little contact with trauma service staff.

Acute trauma is often frightening or upsetting for emergency department staff as well as for those involved in bringing victims to the hospital. Dealing with upset, even distraught, patients and relatives, with those who are acutely disturbed or those who are threatening or violent, makes great demands on clinical skills at all times and especially when departments are busy. While training, experience and a clear clinical role are all important protective factors, the treatment of trauma may in itself be a traumatic experience.

Importance of premorbid mental state and adjustment

There are important ways in which psychiatric disorders and their treatment predispose to trauma (McDonald & Davey, 1996). The presdisposing psychiatric factors are:

(a) substance abuse (alcohol or drugs);
(b) major psychiatric disorder and its treatment;
(c) 'accident-prone personality';
(d) violent behaviour;
(e) delirium;
(f) dementia.

In particular, a history of heavy drinking is extremely common in trauma attenders (Cherpitel, 1993). Pre-existing problems not only increase vulnerability to the range of post-traumatic consequences described later in this chapter, but may well require treatment in their own right, preferably by those who have been previously involved in the patient's care. This will require liaison with all other specialist psychiatric services.

General psychological and social consequences of trauma

The psychological impact of trauma is in many ways similar to that of the other major physical disorders discussed in this book (Table 7.2). Immediate distress is common in those suffering severe or frightening trauma but usually temporary. Persistent anxiety and distress are most likely in those with vulnerable personalities, difficult social circumstances or major continuing medical problems. Effects on everyday functioning are common and persistent (Holbrook *et al*, 1999).

A common and often persistent feature of the emotional reaction to trauma among those who consider they were not at fault is that of *anger* – anger at being an innocent victim and anger at the lack of recognition by those responsible and by others, such as the legal system and insurance companies. We need to be understanding about anger directed elsewhere but also be aware that it may interfere with recovery and treatment.

The trauma may have involved others, unknown to the individual or closely related. The death or injury of relatives or friends, as well as feelings of responsibility and guilt, may greatly increase the overall impact of the trauma. Distress and disability resulting from trauma may have profound consequences for the quality of everyday life of patients and their families and for their financial circumstances. While the main responsibility for offering help lies with social services or in primary care, the assessment of such problems is an essential part of any psychiatric evaluation. Medically unexplained symptoms, such as pain and functional limitation, are quite common.

A very important special feature of trauma is that victims may suffer the psychiatric complications of head injury and specific post-traumatic syndromes. They are also especially likely to suffer

TABLE 7.2
Psychiatric consequences of trauma

Immediate consequences	*Later consequences*
Delirium	Dementia and other cognitive syndromes
Acute stress disorder	Anxiety and depression
Adjustment disorder	Post-traumatic stress disorder
	Post-traumatic phobic anxiety
	Medically unexplained symptoms
	Substance abuse

associated social problems, as well as alcohol and substance abuse. It is important to be aware that many victims are in age groups which are especially financially and socially vulnerable.

Head injury and cognitive disorder

Although head injuries are common, fortunately most are minor and associated with only brief unconsciousness and amnesia, with little evidence of any persistent deficit. In contrast, a very small number are neurologically devastating and require intensive physical and psychiatric rehabilitation with the possibility of long-term care or support. An intermediate group of allegedly minor head injuries cause minor degrees of cognitive impairment, which are often unrecognised by doctors (King, 1997). However, such impairment may cause considerable difficulty in everyday life, both in its own right and in its effects on personality (Kushner, 1998; NIH Consensus Development Panel on Rehabilitation of Persons with Traumatic Brain Injury, 1999).

It is evident that patients with significant head injury require skilled initial medical care and rehabilitation directed towards preventing or treating cognitive, behavioural and/or emotional disturbances and the practical problems of returning to work, social isolation and the burden on carers. The role of the psychiatrist is likely to be modest, especially as clinical psychologists are usually seen as key members of the rehabilitation team. However, the advice of a liaison psychiatrist with neuropsychiatric expertise can be very valuable in the general accident and emergency department, in trauma wards and in specialist regional neurological rehabilitation services.

Specific post-traumatic syndromes

Acute distress often has a mixed picture of anxiety, numbing, dissociation and anger, as well as recurrent memories of the trauma. Some victims report symptoms which satisfy the rather different criteria of acute stress disorder in DSM–IV (American Psychiatric Association, 1994) and ICD–10 (World Health Organization, 1992). Although, fortunately, many of those who suffer immediate distress do not suffer persistent psychiatric complications, an acute syndrome is a predictor of an increased risk of later post-traumatic disorders.

Post-traumatic stress disorder (PTSD) cannot, by convention, be diagnosed until a month after the trauma. It is most likely to occur in relation to particularly frightening accidents and is predicted by some features of early psychological reaction. Prevalence declines over a period of months but a minority of subjects may suffer extremely prolonged and disabling symptoms. Phobic anxiety may be a prominent feature, especially in those involved in transport accidents. It overlaps with the avoidance features of PTSD but often occurs alone and can persist for many years.

Specific aspects of the type of trauma

Road traffic accidents

Road traffic accidents are one of the commonest causes of both major and minor injuries which result in attendance at a trauma unit. Psychological complications after road accidents are as frequent for those who have suffered mild injuries as for those with severe injury. They include depression and anxiety, post-traumatic stress disorder and phobic anxiety about travel. The longer-term occurrence of these complications is difficult to predict in the early days (Mayou *et al*, 1993; Ehlers *et al*, 1998), but evidence of difficulties two to three months after the accident should be seen as indicating the probability of a poor psychosocial outcome. An important subgroup develop post-traumatic stress disorder months or years after the accident. Financial and social problems can be severe for victims and their carers, who may benefit from social work and practical advice.

There is little evidence that preventative debriefing is effective (see below). Current evidence and clinical experience would suggest that supportive measures in the acute phase can proceed in a common-sense way, without major psychiatric input, in the expectation that many problems will improve. Routine advice about return to travel can be helpful. It is then sensible to think of ways in which post-traumatic and other psychiatric problems can be identified and dealt with during convalescence.

Whiplash injury is very common and has attracted particular controversy, especially in relation to the syndrome of neck symptoms and distress and disability, which appears disproportionate to objective medical signs. While frequently dismissed as 'neurotic' or as attributable to simulation or exaggeration, a substantial body of evidence suggests that this is a clearly defined physical syndrome. It is, however, like all road accidents, frequently associated with significant effects on travel and with symptoms of post-traumatic stress disorder. Psychological factors are more important determinants of disability and subjective distress than persistent physical symptoms (Mayou & Bryant, 1996; Mayou & Radanov, 1996).

Domestic injuries

A substantial proportion of injuries happen in the home, from falls, sharp instruments and so on. The elderly are especially likely to suffer falls in which fractures occur, and these often result in hospital admission. Delirium and other psychiatric problems are common and there may be difficulties in arranging appropriate convalescent care. Orthopaedic and trauma wards are very familiar with the difficulties of providing appropriate continuing care for the elderly.

Injury by a spouse, parent, child or other family member will often be a sign of severe family problems, which may require, at the very least, an offer of advice and referral. It may be appropriate to offer or to arrange a place of safety. Legal and ethical issues need to be considered carefully in those instances where victims may be frightened and reluctant to seek help from others. Trauma services obviously need to be aware of these problems and to have clear policies regarding what they do immediately and to what extent help can be made available.

Occupational injuries

Injuries at work are common but usually minor. Occupational health services are expected to be aware of the risks of particular work environments, to take precautions to prevent injury and to minimise the particular risks of those returning to work after an injury. Many studies, especially those relating to back injuries, have indicated that return to work is generally slower after occupational injuries than following similar injuries in other circumstances.

Awareness of occupational issues is important in assessing and treating victims of trauma and especially in writing reports which may affect the timing or the patient's ability to return to work.

Sports injuries

Sports injuries are probably less likely to result in psychological problems than injuries in other circumstances. Even so, experience in specialised sports clinics makes it apparent that inappropriate behaviour and expectations may cause problems in medical management. The psychologist may well have an important role, especially with those who have a professional or very serious amateur involvement.

Assault

Many assaults are physically relatively minor affairs between young men who have often had too much to drink. A few represent serious assault and the police are likely to be involved. Post-traumatic symptoms can be very severe, resulting in stress and marked effects on behaviour.

Sexual assault should always be taken very seriously because of the likelihood of psychological complications and the medico-legal implications. Fortunately, initial emotional distress and the symptoms of post-traumatic stress disorder are often relatively short-lived, but in a substantial minority they can become chronic and have severe effects on everyday life and on relationships. Cognitive–behavioural treatment which includes exposure is effective (Foa *et al*, 1993) and there is encouraging evidence that a brief programme within a month or two of the assault has a marked therapeutic effect on post-traumatic symptoms of depression (Foa *et al*, 1995).

Disasters

Disasters involving many victims have attracted very considerable attention. Disasters may overwhelm individuals, families, communities and health services. There are many causes, which are often divided into natural disasters, such as earthquakes, hurricanes, floods and famine, and man-made disasters, such as transport accidents, crowd incidents, fires, explosions and wars. The psychological consequences may affect victims (survivors, onlookers, relatives), victims by proxy, people who feel responsible for the disaster and a wide range of disaster workers.

The psychological consequences are especially prominent because of the likely severity of the threat, complications from having numbers of victims relating one to another, the practical difficulties of recovery and treatment, and the burden upon those involved in helping and treating victims.

It is generally agreed there is a need for local plans for managing disaster, which enable a rapid, coordinated and expert initial response. While there has been considerable discussion of the role of crisis debriefing, it seems more appropriate to offer initial emotional support with later follow-up to identify complications which may require further specialist intervention (Hobbs *et al*, 1996; Adshead, 1997).

General principles of care

Psychosocial management and the particular role of the liaison psychiatrist follow from an understanding of the immediate problems experienced by a high proportion of victims and others involved and the nature of longer-term psychological complications in a minority. Management comprises, as with the care of all medical problems, the combination of psychologically informed routine medical care by non-specialists together with supervision, training and specialist back-up by psychiatrists, psychologists and social services.

The role of 'debriefing'

There has been a wide assumption that crisis debriefing, focusing on the expression of emotion about the trauma, could have an important, indeed routine, role in care following any frightening trauma. The rationale has been that it not only relieves immediate distress but, more importantly, also prevents the onset of later post-traumatic symptoms. Despite a general acceptance of the rationale and the development of specialist psychiatric services and routine debriefing for those involved in trauma, there is little evidence for its effectiveness (Bisson & Deahl, 1994; Raphael *et al*, 1995; Hobbs *et al*, 1996; Mayou *et al*, 2000). Recent reviews (Wessely *et al*, 1999) and research suggest that debriefing is not effective in its main, prophylactic aim. This is not to deny the value of acute supportive help.

Recognition of chronic post-traumatic problems

The emphasis in managing major post-traumatic psychiatric complications should be on early recognition and individual treatment. Recognition depends on all those involved in medical care being aware of the importance of post-traumatic syndromes, publicising the availability of treatment to victims, lawyers and others who may be involved, and also the inclusion of screening questions in any follow-up assessment.

There are a number of proven treatments. Antidepressant medication is required by those who have clear depressive symptoms, while cognitive–behavioural methods are helpful with those who have persistent post-traumatic stress disorder and the travel problems which are characteristic of road traffic and other transport accidents (Foa and Meadows, 1997; Van Etten and Taylor, 1998).

Special clinical problems

Alcohol problems

Trauma is very frequently associated with alcohol and substance abuse (Cherpitel, 1993). The trauma rarely appears to have a salutary effect on those who have been heavy drinkers and it is not uncommon for drinking to increase, in association with depression, pain and time off work. It should be routine to offer advice on the need to treat such problems and an indication of where help can be obtained. It would be unrealistic to expect such advice to have major benefits but, in a worthwhile number of cases, it may be that the events and trauma do provide an important stimulus to seek help for a chronic problem. Relatively simple forms of help may be effective, especially with less advanced drinking problems (Parish, 1997).

Burns

Premorbid psychiatric problems are especially common in those who suffer major burns. These increase vulnerability to what may have been a very frightening incident, followed by severe pain and medical injuries requiring very prolonged treatment. The psychological and social difficulties of burns patients are usually considerable (Patterson *et al*, 1993). Anxiety and depression are frequent and symptoms of post-traumatic stress disorder have been described in high proportions of subjects.

Spinal injuries

Spinal injuries are fortunately relatively uncommon but require special care and inevitably have profound implications for victims and their families. It is perhaps somewhat surprising that acute distress, depression and anxiety are not more common in the acute stages and that in the longer term most patients achieve a fairly normal mental state rather rapidly (Judd & Brown, 1992; Radnitz *et al*, 1996).

Head injuries

Most head injury is mild but the small proportion of patients who suffer prolonged unconsciousness and amnesia are at high risk of a range of problems. These may be so severe as to require continuing neurological care and rehabilitation, but more often recognition, routine advice and review are most helpful (Eames, 1997). The significance of mild injury should not be underestimated (King, 1997).

There have been several randomised controlled trials of routine case management approaches to reviewing all attendances with head injury and attempting to identify problems early and to make appropriate treatment available. Somewhat surprisingly, these have been ineffective. Considerable clinical input does not seem to have resulted in more effective treatment. There remains a need to consider ways in which all those at risk of any continuing consequences of head injury can be given appropriate advice and medical help.

Cosmetic injuries

Injuries affecting appearance seem to have a particularly profound psychological impact. It is important that victims receive expert plastic surgery assessments at an early stage and that due weight is given to concerns about appearance, which may sometimes seem relatively unimportant to those involved in the patient's care.

Disasters

Disasters affecting relatively small numbers of people can be expected from time to time in any emergency department; major disasters, involving severe injury to many people, are much less common. There is an obvious need for every emergency service to have a medical disaster plan and it should also have a clear plan for the psychological care of patients, relatives and staff (Hobbs, 1995). Increasing clinical experience and research suggest that older ideas concerning some highly potent crisis psychological intervention are unfounded, but there is none the less a great need for policies to ensure that good, clear, supportive care is provided during a time of confusion and distress. The success in providing this will depend upon the whole medical strategy, collecting information and being able to offer follow-up help during recovery.

Care for others involved

Those who suffer physical trauma and who consult or make use of medical services are not the only victims. Bystanders, other participants who are not injured, and relatives and friends who are given upsetting news may also suffer acute distress and be at risk of longer-term post-traumatic symptoms.

The importance of information and advice for relatives is recognised but they are often given unsatisfactorily and this is perhaps particularly true for the acute circumstances of trauma (Cooke *et al*, 1992). Relatives may have been involved in the trauma themselves and be injured; in any case, they are likely to be acutely upset and indeed may be at risk of longer-term psychological complications. Their immediate needs are usually simple. Relatives of those who have been severely injured or who have died in emergency care will require information to be given considerately and in comforting surroundings.

Trauma unit staff and others involved in the care of trauma patients, such as ambulance services, have to confront those with horrific injuries and the considerable stress and suffering of victims and their relatives. Their workload is unpredictable and at times very demanding. Such work makes unpredictable, varied and intense demands on those whose main training has been in physical care. They need appropriate training, supervision and support to ensure that they feel that their work is manageable and worthwhile and that they are doing the best that is possible.

Litigation

The victims of trauma often seek compensation through personal injury claims. Such claims are likely to require medical reports, which increasingly include psychiatric reports. The consultation–liaison psychiatrist may often be asked to describe the psychiatric consequences of trauma and therefore requires knowledge of the common effects of trauma and the skills of writing a clear report.

Most medical and psychiatric literature has tended to emphasise exaggeration and simulation of symptoms among subjects involved in disputed cases; this highly selective experience gives an entirely erroneous impression. A wide range of evidence suggests that involvement in compensation proceedings should be seen as just one of many social factors that may affect the course and outcome following injury (Mendelson, 1995).

Service implications

It would be helpful to have estimates of the size of the clinical problem for psychiatry. Unfortunately, the lack of figures, the great difficulties in comparing workloads between hospitals with different policies in very different types of areas and the lack of psychiatric research make this difficult.

The trauma workload varies very greatly between urban and rural areas. Table 7.3 summarises some relevant points in estimating the immediate and later needs. It is not possible to give precise figures for the frequency of psychological problems or of the proportion of patients who need specialist psychiatric intervention. Although we have important information about the occurrence of problems such as alcohol dependence or post-traumatic stress disorder in some groups, the total size of the clinical problem is unknown and realistic

TABLE 7.3
Points to consider in estimating the clinical needs of trauma victims

Timing	Needs
Immediately	Support and practical help for immediate distress
	Psychiatric referral of deliberate self-harm
	Routine advice concerning possible later post-traumatic problems
	Support and advice for relatives
	Subgroups requiring special attention (victims of rape, burn, spinal injuries)
Later	Specialist advice concerning head injury, major burns, post-traumatic stress disorder, rape, etc.

needs assessment is therefore impossible. None the less, it is certain that the need for psychiatric and psychological services will be substantial in the large general hospital with a busy accident and emergency and trauma service, especially if it also has regional units for problems such as burns and spinal injury. Needs will be much less in the small district general hospital in a rural area in which primary-care services may be more actively involved in continuing care.

Review of the psychological implications of trauma and of common problems enables us to consider the possible contribution by the liaison psychiatrist based in a general hospital. In practice, the liaison psychiatrist should begin by aiming to meet conspicuous demands from colleagues, by establishing a working relationship in which the size of the clinical need can be identified and in which a start can be made on the supervision and training of trauma unit medical and nursing staff and providing a good emergency consultation service.

It is necessary to consider a number of practical issues:

(a) the place of consultation (hospital emergency department, accident in-patient unit, primary care, workplace);
(b) its timing after the trauma (immediate, early or late)
(c) the nature of the clinical problem (see Table 7.3).

Table 7.4 sets out elements for a service which provides emergency consultation. There is a clear role for the liaison psychiatrist to be seen as providing a centre of expertise which is available to give advice and help to others, whether they work in the hospital, in primary care or elsewhere. Finally, the liaison psychiatrist has an important role in giving advice on the support for staff, which should be constructive and focused rather than overly ambitious.

TABLE 7.4

Elements of a service providing consultation–liaison to a trauma unit

Main elements	Specific concerns
Twenty-four hour emergency department and in-patient consultation	
Liaison with other psychiatric services, social workers, and community and voluntary groups with regard to continuing care and review	
Training and supervision for trauma unit and other staff	Acute distress Distress of relatives Post-traumatic symptoms Head injury Substance abuse Disturbed behaviour Deliberate self-harm Rape, domestic violence
Support for staff	
Access to specialist out-patient clinic	Urgent and routine referral
Disaster planning	
Centre of psychiatric expertise	Advice, assessment and treatment Training Supervision

Psychological care for trauma in the emergency department

How can a trauma service meet these needs? Since trauma units are substantially part of emergency departments, these needs have to be considered against the wider needs of all emergency attenders, which may include a wide range of psychiatric problems. This means that psychiatric, social and other services for *trauma* are most efficiently organised as part of a wider emergency department liaison (Table 7.4). A 24-hour presence in the emergency department and availability in the in-patient wards may seem desirable and, indeed, in very large hospitals, possible. However, it is more important to concentrate on procedures for enabling emergency department staff to provide the highest possible care themselves, training them to recognise problems and then to make more specialist psychiatric skills available in ways that are feasible and are acceptable for patients.

Help is likely to be best provided by a multi-disciplinary team of medical, nursing and other staff who have particular experience of the emergency department and good working relationships. The list in Table 7.4 shows that a substantial contribution can come from training, supervision and close liaison with trauma unit staff. This could give nursing, medical and other staff the expertise and confidence to deal with many routine problems and to recognise those who may need extra assistance, either as an emergency referral or from early attendance at a specialist referral clinic.

Specialist psychological services for trauma

The evidence on types of trauma and types of clinical problem reviewed above indicates that small proportions of trauma patients have special psychological needs, which may continue over long periods. A few of these will be in-patients, but most will be at home. These needs are unlikely to be met by community-based psychiatry services whose expertise and interest in these areas is limited. The most efficient and effective alternative is the development of a specialist service offering assessment and treatment. It is likely to require psychiatric, psychological and social expertise and will be most effective if it is closely coordinated with the trauma service itself.

The specialist post-traumatic stress disorder clinic

A few specialist clinics have been established in a number of countries to offer treatment to trauma victims with severe post-traumatic symptoms. Some of these clinics have special interests in particular forms of trauma, such as rape, assault and combat. Clinics and procedures have also been established in the workplace and in other special settings. There has been no rationale behind these ventures, which have almost always been in response to a particular conspicuous need or have developed from a specialised research programme. Few of these services have had links with consultation–liaison psychiatry.

Audit and evaluation

Since psychiatric services to trauma units are in their infancy, audit and evaluation must be directed to demonstrating clinical needs as well as describing the impact of new psychiatric and other services.

Conclusions

The psychiatric issues in relation to trauma are in many ways similar to the specialist medical and surgical services ones. There are, however, special issues in relation to the psychiatric consequences of trauma and in relation to the best ways of delivering care to potentially large numbers of trauma victims, most of whom are seen only briefly for their medical problems but who may suffer severe and persistent psychological disturbance. Psychiatric care for the victims of trauma is haphazard and has not as yet been a major theme in consultation–liaison psychiatry. This chapter has highlighted both the scale of the problem and the scope for better care. It has, above all, argued that the expertise of consultation–liaison psychiatry is needed in this area, although it still requires substantial development, and should be applied to the provision of expertise based substantially within the general hospital but offering flexible, specialist advice and treatment services for both the immediate and later clinical problems.

This chapter provides an outline for psychiatric services directed to those with acute trauma attending accident and emergency departments, as well as other, more specialised, medical and surgical services, and also for those presenting or being followed up in primary care. It is a model which needs to be presented to purchasers and others involved in planning as offering significant help to large numbers of distressed and disabled people, people who, in hospital and primary care, are currently responsible for a very large proportion of health service direct costs, as well as very large indirect costs.

The liaison psychiatrist who understands the different types of traumas and their medical and psychological complications, related clinical problems, and how they are managed within the emergency department, other hospital services and in primary care, will be able to devise services which offer informed and flexible psychiatric consultation and more general advice, supervision and training. The ultimate success of any initiative depends upon greater understanding of the psychological impact of trauma in both specialist and general practice care, and in the general population. General acceptance of the psychological impact of trauma, awareness of the resilience of most victims and the normality of a number of unpleasant and disabling symptoms should enable us to develop a combination of supportive routine care with a targeting of specialist procedures upon those most in need and most likely to benefit.

References

ADSHEAD, G. (1997) Psychological services for road accident victims and their relatives. In *The aftermath of road accidents. Psychological, social and legal consequences of an everyday trauma* (ed. M. Mitchell), pp. 217–223. London: Routledge.

AMERICAN PSYCHIATRIC ASSOCIATION (1994) *Diagnostic and Statistical Manual of Mental Disorders* (4th edn) (DSM–IV). Washington, DC: APA.

BISSON, J. I. & DEAHL, M. P. (1994) Psychological debriefing and prevention of post-traumatic stress. More research is needed. *British Journal of Psychiatry*, **165**, 717–720.

BURDETT-SMITH, P. (1992) Estimating trauma centre workload. *Journal of the Royal College of Surgeons, Edinburgh*, **37**, 128–130.

CHERPITEL, C. J. (1993) Alcohol and injuries: a review of international emergency room studies. *Addiction*, **88**, 923–937.

COOKE, M. W., COOKE, H. M. & GLUCKSMAN, E. E. (1992) Management of sudden bereavement in the accident and emergency department. *British Medical Journal*, **304**, 1207–1209.

DRISCOLL, P. A. (1992) Trauma: today's problems, tomorrow's answers. *Injury*, **23**, 151–158.

EAMES, P. (1997) Traumatic brain injury. *Current Opinion in Psychiatry*, **10**, 49–52.

EHLERS, A., MAYOU, R. & BRYANT, B. (1998) Psychological predictors of chronic PTSD after motor vehicle accidents. *Journal of Abnormal Psychology*, **107**, 508–519.

EVANS, R. C. & EVANS, R. J. (1992) Reviews in medicine. *Accident and Emergency Postgraduate Medical Journal*, **68**, 714–734, 786–793.

FOA, E. B., ROTHBAUM, B. O. & STEKETEE, G. S. (1993) Treatment of rape victims. *Journal of Interpersonal Violence*, **8**, 256–276.

——, HEARST-IKEDA, D. & PERRY, K. J. (1995) Evaluation of a brief cognitive–behavioural program for the prevention of chronic PTSD in recent assault victims. *Journal of Consulting and Clinical Psychology*, **63**, 948–955.

—— & MEADOWS, E. A. (1997) Psychological treatments for posttraumatic stress disorder: a critical review. *Annual Review of Psychology*, **48**, 449–480.

HOBBS, M. (1995) A district framework for managing psychosocial aspects of disaster. *Advances in Psychiatric Treatment*, **1**, 176–183.

——, Mayou, R., Harrison, B., *et al* (1996) A randomised controlled trial of psychological debriefing for victims of road traffic accidents. *British Medical Journal*, **313**, 1438–1439.

HOLBROOK, T. L., ANDERSON, J. P., SIEBER, W. J., *et al* (1999) Outcome after major trauma: 12-month and 18-month follow-up results from the Trauma Recovery Project. *Journal of Trauma: Injury, Infection and Critical Care*, **46**, 765–773.

JUDD, F. K. & BROWN, D. J. (1992) Psychiatric consultation in a spinal injuries unit. *Australian and New Zealand Journal of Psychiatry*, **26**, 218–222.

KING, N. (1997) Literature review. Mild head injury: neuropathology, sequelae, measurement and recovery. *British Journal of Clinical Psychology*, **36**, 161–184.

KUSHNER, D. (1998) Mild traumatic brain injury: toward understanding manifestations and treatment. *Archives of Internal Medicine*, **158**, 1617–1624.

MAYOU, R., BRYANT, B. & DUTHIE, R. (1993) Psychiatric consequences of road traffic accidents. *British Medical Journal*, **307**, 647–651.

—— & BRYANT, B. (1996) Outcome of "whiplash" neck injury. *Injury*, **27**, 617–623.

—— & RADANOV, B. P. (1996) Whiplash neck injury. *Journal of Psychosomatic Research*, **40**, 461–474.

——, EHLERS, A. & HOBBS, M. (2000) Psychological debriefing for road traffic accident victims. Three-year follow-up of a randomised controlled trial. *British Journal of Psychiatry*, **176**, 589–593.

MCDONALD, A. S. & DAVEY, G. C. L. (1996) Psychiatric disorders and accidental injury. *Clinical Psychology Review*, **16**, 105–127.

MENDELSON, G. (1995) "Compensation neurosis" revisited: outcome studies of the effects of litigation. *Journal of Psychosomatic Research*, **39**, 695–706.

NIH CONSENSUS DEVELOPMENT PANEL ON REHABILITATION OF PERSONS WITH TRAUMATIC BRAIN INJURY (1999) Rehabilitation of persons with traumatic brain injury. *Journal of the American Medical Association*, **282**, 974–983.

PARISH, D. C. (1997) Another indication for screening and early intervention: problem drinking. *Journal of the American Medical Association*, **277**, 1079–1080.

PATTERSON, D. R., EVERETT, J. J., BOMBARDIER, C. H., *et al* (1993) Psychological effects of severe burn injuries. *Psychological Bulletin*, **113**, 362–378.

RADNITZ, C. L., BRODERICK, C. P., PEREZ-STRUMOLO, L., *et al* (1996) The prevalence of psychiatric disorders in veterans with spinal cord injury: a controlled comparison. *Journal of Nervous and Mental Disease*, **184**, 431–433.

RAPHAEL, B., MELDRUM, L. & MCFARLANE, A. C. (1995) Does debriefing after psychological trauma work? *British Medical Journal*, **310**, 1479–1480.

VAN ETTEN, M. L. & TAYLOR, S. (1998) Comparative efficacy of treatments for post-traumatic stress disorder: a meta-analysis. *Clinical Psychology and Psychotherapy*, **5**, 126–144.

WESSELY, S., ROSE, S. & BISSON, J. (1999) A systematic review of brief psychological interventions ("debriefing") for the treatment of immediate trauma related symptoms and the prevention of post traumatic stress disorder (Cochrane Review). *Cochrane Library*, Issue 4. Oxford: Software Update.

WORLD HEALTH ORGANIZATION (1992) *International Classification of Diseases and Related Health Problems* (10th edn) (ICD–10). Geneva: WHO.

8   Liaison psychiatry in the pain clinic

CHRISTOPHER BASS

Most district general hospitals in the UK have a multi-disciplinary pain clinic, staffed by anaesthetists, psychologists, nurses, physiotherapists and occupational therapists. Some have in-patient beds, and some offer a service for patients with postoperative pain as well as a range of chronic painful disorders. In general hospitals that have access to liaison psychiatry services, important links can be forged between the liaison psychiatrist and the pain clinic (Dolin & Stephens, 1998).

This chapter begins with a description of the organisation and planning of psychiatry services to a pain clinic, the prevalence and nature of psychiatric morbidity in pain clinic populations and the sources of referral. Methods of assessing these patients are also described. This is followed by a discussion of management strategies for patients with chronic pain and 'models' of working with colleagues from other disciplines. Emphasis is on clinical practice rather than detailed explanations of empirical research. Reference is made, however, to key research papers in the field and wherever possible randomised controlled studies are cited.

Organisation and planning

The planners of health services have been slow to recognise the importance of providing psychological and psychiatric services to general hospital pain clinics. This is surprising, given the high rates of psychiatric morbidity in these samples (see below).

Most pain clinics in the UK are organised by anaesthetists. Referrals are accepted from other hospital specialists as well as from local general practitioners. A proportion of referrals also come from

The pain clinic   93

outside the region. A clinical psychologist is an essential component of any multi-disciplinary pain team, and many have full-time clinical attachments to pain clinics.

Very few psychiatric services have established links with pain clinics; most psychiatric services have to respond to increasing demands from the community and have little time and few resources to liaise with pain clinics. Because a high proportion of patients referred to the liaison psychiatrist report acute or chronic pain, and some of these may have already established contact with pain clinic services, it is important for the liaison psychiatrist to establish a good working relationship with the pain clinic (see later). This liaison may involve a number of fixed clinical sessions or a working relationship with the pain clinicians. Before this is established, however, it is important to set up appropriate funding arrangements between the finance departments of the relevant hospital trusts.

Whatever working arrangement is established with the pain clinic, liaison psychiatrists should be aware of their limitations and not be 'swamped' by referrals. The management of patients with chronic pain therefore depends not only on the resources within the liaison psychiatry team (including psychologists, nurses and occupational therapists), but also on the ability of the local community mental health teams to provide additional help, as well as on the resources available in primary care.

Prevalence of psychiatric morbidity in pain clinic populations

Until recently, few studies had examined both the psychiatric and the physical status of patients attending pain clinics. Benjamin et al (1988) examined relationships between chronic pain, organic disease and mental illness in a UK regional pain relief unit. Of the 106 consecutive patients assessed using standardised psychiatric interviews, approximately half had diagnosed mental illness and two-thirds organic disease. Pain ratings were higher in those with mental illness but were *not* related to the presence of organic pathology. The key finding was that there was no evidence that the subjects could be simply divided into those with physical and those with mental illness.

A similar high rate of psychiatric illness was reported in patients admitted to a North American in-patient pain unit. Katon et al (1985) found that the most frequent psychiatric diagnoses were major depression (32% were in a current episode and 43% had recorded a past episode) and alcohol abuse (41%). More than half the patients had a history of one or more episodes of major depression or alcohol abuse before the onset of their chronic pain. Such high rates of alcohol abuse are unlikely to be present in an equivalent British pain sample, although Kouyanou *et al* (1997*a*) found that psychoactive substance abuse or dependence was diagnosed in 12% of patients with chronic pain attending a South London pain clinic.

In another North American study, of 283 consecutive admissions to a university pain centre, anxiety syndromes and depression of various types were the most frequently assigned axis I diagnoses, with over half the patient sample receiving each of these diagnoses (Fishbain *et al*, 1986). Males were significantly over-represented among those diagnosed with intermittent explosive disorders, adjustment disorders with work inhibitions and alcohol and drug abuse, whereas females were significantly over-represented among those with current depression and somatoform disorders. In this study 58% of patients also fulfilled criteria for personality disorders, with dependent (17%), passive–aggressive (15%) and histrionic (12%) patterns being the most frequent.

The high concordance of physical and psychological disorders in pain clinic populations has also been reported in primary care. Pain conditions are common in the general population and the presence of multiple chronic pain symptoms is associated with elevated levels of anxiety, depression, non-pain physical symptoms and less favourable health appraisal (Dworkin *et al*, 1990). Croft *et al* (1993) found a prevalence of chronic widespread pain in the general population of 11.2%. In view of these important research findings, it is evident that psychological services should be readily available in pain clinics. Whether these services are provided by clinical psychology or liaison psychiatry is often determined by local factors, but ideally there should be a contribution from both disciplines.

Sources of referral

In practice, liaison psychiatrists receive referrals from colleagues in pain clinics. In many cases psychological problems will have become evident during an in-patient stay and impeded conventional medical treatment. Alternatively, an out-patient will be referred for an assessment. The liaison psychiatrist may either be asked for an opinion regarding some aspects of treatment or be requested to take over the management of the patient.

The liaison psychiatry service may also receive referrals of patients with chronic pain indirectly, via the deliberate self-harm service, that is, from the accident and emergency department. Some large district general hospitals have designated services for these patients, some of whom take drug overdoses because of chronic, intractable pain. It is important to recall that certain physical illnesses are associated with higher than average rates of suicide (Harris & Barraclough, 1994) and that age-adjusted suicide completion rates for patients experiencing chronic pain are significantly greater than those of the general population (Fishbain *et al*, 1991). Some patients with chronic pain who deliberately harm themselves are very difficult to help; this is illustrated in the following case vignette.

A 65-year-old woman was seen in the short-stay ward of our hospital after taking 40 co-proxamol tablets. She complained of "constant back pain for 18 years" which was "unbearable agony". This had provoked the overdose, which was of low suicidal intent but medically dangerous. She had been investigated on numerous previous occasions by orthopaedic and rheumatological specialists but no relevant organic disease had been detected on either computed tomography or magnetic resonance imaging scans. There were no abnormal physical signs apart from limitation of lumbar flexion caused by spasm in the paraspinal muscles.

She had not worked for over 20 years and had consulted numerous other specialists, both in the private and complementary sectors. She remained convinced of an organic cause for her pain, a view shared by her doting husband, who had given up his job, spent all his savings on his wife's illness and colluded with her illness beliefs.

She reported a history of recurrent depression and alcohol abuse, but the severity of the back pain (uncharacteristically) bore no relation to her mood disorder. At interview the most obvious abnormality was her distress, abnormal illness beliefs and pain behaviours. She was referred to the psychogeriatric service, where a plan was made to manage the family systemically in an attempt to help the patient (and her family) cope with and manage the pain and reduce their expectations of cure.

Components of psychological assessment

In order to receive appropriate referrals from pain clinic colleagues, good relations are essential. These can be built up only by providing what is perceived to be a good service over time. A referrer should make it clear to the patient that pain has a psychological dimension and that both physical and psychological factors are important to assess in conditions characterised by chronic pain. It is also important for the referrer to state explicitly that the patient is going to see a psychiatrist: bland statements such as "a colleague with an interest in emotional problems" is not acceptable.

There are some clinical indicators that suggest that psychosocial factors are important in chronic pain, and one or more may prompt referral for psychiatric assessment (Sullivan *et al*, 1991). These are:

(a) the pain persists beyond healing time;
(b) a disparity between objective findings and functional disability;
(c) an excessive use of health care services;
(d) signs or symptoms of psychiatric disorder;
(e) prolonged or excessive use of opiates, benzodiazepines, or alcohol.

Whenever possible, pain colleagues should be prompted to refer *early* rather than after a series of normal investigations and/or failed therapeutic procedures.

A suggested method of preparing a patient for referral to a psychiatrist is as follows:

"Your symptoms of pain are very real but I think that psychological and emotional difficulties may be making a contribution to your physical problems at present. It is as important to address the psychological problems as it is to deal with the physical ones. I have a colleague, Dr X, a psychiatrist, who has a particular interest in patients like you. Dr X works in the general hospital (not in a psychiatric hospital) and has had a lot of experience helping patients with problems like yours. Would you like me to arrange an appointment for you to see Dr X?"

The initial interview

The objectives the initial assessment are as follows:

(a) to clarify the patient's complaints – to gain an understanding of why this particular person became ill in this particular way at this particular time;
(b) to understand what the patient wants;
(c) to elicit fears and beliefs about the pain;
(d) to elicit the contribution of *relevant* organic disease to the patient's pain complaints;
(e) to identify the relevant psychosocial stressors (antecedent and current);
(f) to identify salient maintaining factors (see below);
(g) to identify psychiatric disorder (or relevant psychophysiological processes; such as hyperventilation or increased muscle tension).

This cannot always be accomplished in a single interview, since the patient with chronic pain may have mixed or even frankly hostile feelings towards the idea of seeing a psychiatrist. It is important to accept the physical symptoms as real and a sensible way to start is by asking patients what the referring physician (often the pain clinic doctor) has told them about the reasons for referral. This can be followed by an enquiry about patients' attitudes towards seeing a psychiatrist, perhaps mentioning that most people would naturally be apprehensive and possibly feel stigmatised. It is essential to be clear at the outset about whether patients feel angry at the referral or, in patients where physical investigations have ruled out disease, continue strongly to believe that their symptoms are due to a still undiagnosed physical disease (House, 1995).

Thereafter, is advisable to proceed with the interview in a sequence which begins with the physical complaints of pain and moves on to psychological topics as the interview progresses. A suggested sequence is therefore:

(a) attitude to referral;
(b) pain details;
(c) effect on daily life (disability);
(d) previous experience of doctors/treatment;
(e) illness history (self and family);
(f) developmental history;
(g) history of emotional distress;
(h) current beliefs/attitudes about pain;
(i) current distress and mental state;
(j) rating scales;
(k) formulation of problem.

A chronological account of the current physical complaints is the natural starting point; this will include the various contacts with the referring and other doctors, treatments received and their effects. Then ask about any disability, limitations of activity or avoidance. This allows patients to talk about any losses, for example in their work or leisure activities, and may provide an opportunity to respond to mood cues.

During this part of the interview, negative interaction with one or more doctors is frequently disclosed. This should be explored, the patient given the opportunity to ventilate, and appropriate empathic statements made. Enquiries should be made about any physical illness in the parents, perhaps leading to parental invalidism, for example. If so, further enquiries should focus on how the family coped with pain and illness and what the impact of these illnesses was on the patient. This overlaps with a personal history; particular enquiry should be made about attitudes to illness in the family during the patient's upbringing (Gill & Bass, 1997; Barsky, 1998). Some patients may have had physical illnesses as a child and it is important to ask what kinds of illness, whether these led to any hospital admissions, how the parents reacted and coped, what was the child told about the illness (e.g. whether it was necessary to avoid sport and physical exercise), what incapacity resulted and whether the illness led to any prolonged school absences. It is also important to ask whether any previous episodes of illness were linked to life events, what procedures, if any, were undertaken and what were the findings.

After these issues have been discussed (and the patient has the right not to talk about them) it is often easier to explore more emotional aspects of the history and to ask about any past episodes of psychological illness.

The interview should end with a mental state examination with particular emphasis on beliefs and attitudes about the symptoms as well as attitudes to the medical profession and to health and illness generally. Pain beliefs and attitudes can be measured with rating scales (see below), and questions should be asked about symptom attributions, reasons (if any) for holding strong conviction of disease despite evidence to the contrary, and the worst fears associated with the pain.

Current mood should be assessed, with specific attention paid to vegetative symptoms of depression, panic and anxiety. It is important to ask about any psychotropic or other drug use, and to quantify the amount of analgesic and psychotropic drugs taken during the day. Asking about a typical day, with the patient describing details of pain and behaviour on an hourly basis throughout the day, is often helpful and may provide further evidence of disability. It is also important to ask routinely about the use of alcohol and prescribed medication, as well as over-the-counter (non-prescribed) drugs.

Assessment of pain behaviours

Patients display a range of reactions to pain, some of which are observable. These have been called pain behaviours, which are important in there own right not only because they can be observed and quantified, but also because they elicit responses from others (Turk & Okifuji, 1999). Common overt pain behaviours are shown in Table 8.1. Pain behaviours can also become a habitual pattern through various types of social reinforcement, such as attention, avoidance of undesirable activities and financial compensation.

TABLE 8.1
Pain behaviours

Categories	Behaviours
Verbal/vocalisation	Sighs, moans Repeated complaints
Motor	Facial grimacing Distorted gait (limping) Rigid or unstable posture Excessively slow or laboured movement
Seek help/reduce pain	Take medication Use of protective device (crutches, cervical collar, wheelchair) Visit doctor
Functional limitation	Resting Reduced activity

Adapted from Turk & Okifuji (1999).

Learned pain behaviours should not be mistaken for malingering. Malingering is the conscious and purposeful faking of a symptom to achieve some benefit, usually financial. Most patients who display learned pain behaviours are not aware of doing so, nor are they consciously motivated to obtain positive reinforcement with the behaviours, whereas malingering patients may intentionally exhibit exaggerated behaviours indicative of pain. However, there is very little evidence that outright faking of pain for financial gain is widespread. The assessment should document those factors that increase or decrease pain behaviours. Such behaviours can also be observed when a patient is in the waiting room and being escorted to the interview room, during an interview, and/or during a series of structured tasks.

Use of standard rating scales

It is often helpful at this stage to use rating scales in an attempt to quantify the physical and psychological symptoms. The Hospital Anxiety and Depression Scale (Zigmond & Snaith, 1983) and the Whiteley Index (Pilowsky, 1967) are particularly helpful, as are more 'psychological' questionnaires such as the Pain Cognitions Questionnaire (Boston *et al*, 1990) and the Survey of Patient Attitudes – which measures beliefs (Jensen *et al*, 1987). The Illness Perception Questionnaire also yields important information about the patient's beliefs and expectations (Weinman *et al*, 1996). An attempt should be made to assess the patient's coping strategies (Rosenstiel & Keefe, 1983) because these may have a bearing on outcome. Common strategies include distraction, ignoring pain sensations, reinterpreting pain, catastrophising, and praying and hoping (Swartzman *et al*, 1994). Finally, it is useful to have a baseline rating of the patient's level of functional disability, and this can be achieved by using the short-form 36 Health Survey Questionnaire (Ware & Sherbourne, 1992) or the Global Assessment of Functioning Scale (Phelan *et al*, 1994), or both. A good review of the various problems posed in the measurement of pain has been published (Skevington, 1995).

Formulation of the problem

Assessment may take more than one appointment. The interviewer should try to produce a formulation, distinguishing between pre-disposing, precipitating and maintaining factors. Management must focus on the last, which may include disparate factors:

(a) depression, anxiety and panic disorder;
(b) dependent or avoidant personality disorder;
(c) chronic marital and/or interpersonal discord;
(d) occupational factors;
(e) iatrogenic factors (e.g. over-investigation);
(f) abnormal illness beliefs (in patient *and* family);
(g) chronic inactivity, leading to muscle wasting;
(h) compensation, litigation and benefits.

It is also important to interview any carers, partners or spouses for their opinions about the pain. Indeed, it is advisable to involve the patients' relatives in the management plan from the outset; this may reduce the risk of early relapse after discharge from an in-patient pain treatment unit (Benjamin *et al*, 1992; see also the case vignette above).

Preparing the patient for psychological treatment

Before treatment is begun, there are three important issues:

(a) All investigations should have been completed; the patient should be told that the treatment is conditional on no further investigations being carried out.
(b) The patient should be informed that a pain- or symptom-free existence may not be a realistic therapeutic goal; for most patients it will be more appropriate to help them cope better with their pain and disability, that is, 'coping not curing'.

(c) The nature of the treatment and its approximate duration should be carefully explained. It is important for the patient to be 'engaged' in treatment and to be involved in the collaborative therapeutic process.

The aims and goals of treatment should be made explicit from the outset. Some patients have chronic, intractable problems that are unlikely to respond to a brief, focused, psychological approach.

Treatments

The treatment approaches can be divided into psychological treatment, which includes cognitive–behavioural therapy, behaviour therapy and psychodynamic psychotherapy (Guthrie *et al*, 1991), and pharmacological treatment. The choice of depends, to a large extent, on the orientation of the psychiatrist and the way in which the formulation is made. For example, a cognitive–behavioural formulation will lead naturally to a therapeutic approach that tackles dysfunctional beliefs and abnormal behaviour, such as spending 20 hours a day in bed and avoiding exercise. Such patients would not only be asked about their illness beliefs and assumptions – and encouraged to provide alternative explanations for these – but also asked to carry out graded exercise, in particular gradually increasing periods out of bed. This treatment approach has been described in more detail elsewhere (Sharpe, 1995).

Some clinical characteristics have a bearing on the type of treatment to be used. For example, marked behavioural abnormalities suggest that behavioural treatment may be more appropriate, whereas cognitive treatment may be better suited to a patient with dysfunctional beliefs about pain. It is often appropriate to prescribe tricyclic antidepressants, which have been shown to have analgesic effects that are independent of their antidepressant effect (McQuay & Moore, 1997). In practice, the available treatments are not discrete; indeed, there is considerable overlap, and the type of treatment can be modified according to the needs (and assessment) of each patient (Table 8.2).

Many patients wrongly believe that antidepressants are addictive. Tell the patient that the antidepressants are in fact misnamed, and have multiple actions on many systems of the body. It is often helpful to explain that the same chemical messages that go awry in depression are known to be involved in part of the pain pathway. So-called side-effects can actually be very helpful, with sedative properties helping with anxiety and insomnia. Even the atropinic effects can be an

TABLE 8.2
Flexible management of chronic pain

Type of management	Specific interventions
Symptom oriented	Relaxation Antidepressant drugs
Behaviourally oriented	Reducing inappropriate use of health services
Function oriented	Pain management Graded increase in activity
Aetiologically oriented	Cognitive therapy Psychodynamic therapy
Containment and support	Limit patient expectations of cure

advantage in some cases, for example in irritable bowel syndrome with marked abdominal pain.

Occupational and social factors

The workplace may be a source of both psychological and physical stress and changes in working practice may be important in the management of musculoskeletal pain and other chronic painful disorders. Negotiation with occupational physicians or with the patient's employers can therefore be important in achieving a return to work. Problems with the return to work because of dissatisfaction with employment is a major potential obstacle to rehabilitation (Hotopf, 1998). A gradual return to full duties is extremely helpful, to which some employers – not usually including the National Health Service – are sympathetic.

The need for flexibility

Flexibility in treatment is essential (see Table 8.2). Separate therapeutic techniques may have to be used, depending on the nature of the maintaining factors. For example, in some patients undergoing cognitive–behavioural therapy, an intrusive marital problem may emerge which requires the introduction of marital or family therapy.

It is easy to lose sight of the fact that change may be very gradual and that the treatment process may last for as long as six months or possibly years. "Broadening the agenda" (Goldberg *et al*, 1989) to involve discussion of psychosocial issues in chronic pain patients is a long-term undertaking and it is often easy for the therapist to lose sight of the treatment gains (or losses). This underscores the need for mutually agreed and realistic treatment aims and goals.

A long-term strategy is required for a subgroup of patients with chronic, enduring pain characterised by high somatic awareness linked with a predisposition to develop physical symptoms at times of stress. Such patients, many of whom satisfy criteria for somatisation disorder, may require long-term supportive, empathic management designed to improve self-esteem and self-efficacy (Bass, 1996). In such cases, it is unclear who should manage the patient and for how long: should it be the responsibility of the general practitioner, hospital doctor, or psychiatrist, or should the general practitioner manage the patient with advice and support from the psychiatrist? Sometimes the pain clinic can offer a useful place for such patients to be contained and managed, as illustrated in the case vignette below.

A 33-year-old woman was referred while receiving treatment as an in-patient in the regional pain clinic. She reported constant pain in her right groin for the last two years. She also reported symptoms suggestive of irritable bowel syndrome.

She had a very disturbed background and was raped at the age of 17. She married at 18 and had two children. This was followed by dyspareunia and menorrhagia, for which she had a hysterectomy at the age of 25. She felt coerced into having the hysterectomy and after this reported constant lower abdominal pain. Three years after this she had another operation with division of adhesions and since that time she had had more right-sided abdominal pain, which extended into the right groin. She also had symptoms of bloating and distension, with altered bowel habit, which complicated the presentation.

She reported panic attacks after the birth of both children, and examination of her general practice file revealed episodes of chest, neck and facial pain in the previous 10 years, for which no organic cause had been found.

Her description of a typical pain day revealed very limited activity, preoccupation with the pain and a lot of resting and lying down. She was unable to work because of the pain and did only a minimal amount of housework.

In summary, this 33-year-old woman had longstanding problems with multiple unexplained pain syndromes and dyspareunia and menstrual irregularities which led to a hysterectomy at the aged of 25. After this she had had chronic abdominal pain for which another operation had failed to provide relief. Her abdominal complaints were complicated by symptoms of irritable bowel syndrome and the interview revealed a hostility and lack of trust towards doctors.

At interview it was clear that she had not come to terms with either the rape or the menstrual irregularities and how these had been dealt with by the medical profession. A management plan was outlined which involved no further invasive procedures and an agreement was made with the patient that she would deal with some of the psychological issues that had been troubling her in the past. She was seen by a female psychiatrist at regular, fixed intervals over the course of the next three years. During that time she had no further medical investigations or operations, learned to cope with and manage her pain with less disability, and became less disabled. She also acquired a voluntary job working as a secretary and her mood improved with 100 mg amitriptyline.

Role of the liaison psychiatrist in the pain clinic

The importance of establishing good relationships with members of the pain clinic staff has already been emphasised. This includes establishing links with nurses on the in-patient unit (if such a resource is available), the receptionist, psychologists, occupational therapists and pain consultants. Many psychologists who work in pain clinics establish, and are involved in the day-to-day running of, out-patient pain-management groups, usually for up to eight patients. This is an important resource, as the referral of some patients to such a pain-management programme may be appropriate. In our trust, the liaison psychiatrist refers patients to and receives patients from the out-patient pain management group. It is important for the liaison psychiatrist to be aware of the clinical and other indications for referral to such an out-patient pain-management programme:

(a) the pain is localised, not in multiple sites, although this indication should not be regarded as absolute;
(b) there is no gross personality disorder or mental illness;
(c) there is no drug or alcohol misuse;
(d) the patient is motivated to improve;
(e) there are supportive relatives;
(f) there are no transport problems;
(g) the patient is willing to work in a group;
(h) the patient is able to communicate.

The local pain clinic may also be the site of other specialised clinics for patients with circumscribed problems such as headache or facial pain. Again, it is important to discover where these clinics are held, who administers them and the type of clinical problem accepted by the receiving clinicians.

The joint pain clinic

In certain instances it may be appropriate to review a patient's pain problem in a joint clinic. In the author's experience, such a clinic can be particularly helpful in those patients in whom the psychological contribution to symptoms and disability is complex, such as those with trivial joint disease who become grossly disabled and attract a diagnosis of fibromyalgia, or patients who after a technically successful operation for angina (coronary artery bypass graft surgery) continue to report disabling non-cardiac chest pain one year after surgery. Such clinics offer a number of distinct advantages and these are discussed under separate headings below.

Minimising stigma

Patients who would be stigmatised by a referral to the psychiatric service may find it more acceptable to be referred to a pain clinic with both a psychiatrist and a pain specialist present (it is, of course, imperative for the patient to be informed before referral to such a clinic that a psychiatrist will be present at the interview!).

Sharing clinical information

The pain clinician may prescribe a medication with which the psychiatrist is unfamiliar, or be able to discuss the relevance of certain physical test results such as a magnetic resonance imaging scan in a patient with back pain. By contrast, the psychiatrist may be able to highlight the contribution of a key maintaining factor in chronic pain such as unresolved grief, depression, markedly abnormal illness beliefs or iatrogenic factors (Kouyanou *et al*, 1997*b*; see also above). Reassurance proffered by the pain specialist about a negative or equivocal test is also likely to be more powerful in such a setting than if given by a psychiatrist alone.

Educational opportunities

The joint clinic holds opportunities for educating the patient about the pain experience and factors that influence this. The patient also learns that both physical *and* psychological factors are important maintaining factors in chronic pain. Furthermore, both pain clinician and psychiatrist have the opportunity to learn from each other, and the clinical psychologist will provide additional insights into the contribution and relevance of certain pain beliefs and behaviours as well as psychological treatment techniques. The joint clinic also provides an excellent and important opportunity for the education of junior medical staff, including both anaesthetists and psychiatrists in training.

Case conferences

Patients who are heavy users of medical services often have coexisting psychological problems. Many different clinicians may be involved in a fruitless attempt to bring about a 'cure' in a patient who is making unrealistic and unreasonable demands (Sharpe *et al*, 1994). It is often appropriate to arrange a case conference for the patient (and family) and to invite the various clinicians involved in the patient's care to discuss and implement a mutually agreed management plan. The pain clinic is often the optimum location for such a case conference, being both in the general hospital and psychologically 'neutral'. At such conferences it is often appropriate to introduce the patient to the idea that management will be gradually shifted from a predominantly 'biomedical' to a 'psychosocial' framework of care, involving containment and support rather than further surgery and physical investigations (see Fig. 1). An example of such a conference follows.

A 40-year-old amputee was referred from the orthopaedic in-patient ward after expressing suicidal ideas to the nursing staff. A previously active, energetic electrician, he had injured his right leg four years previously by falling off a ladder. As a consequence of this accident his knee had become so unstable that he required an above-knee amputation. Unfortunately, he continued to report pain in the stump and, as a result of chronic infection, required two revisions of the stump in the next three years. The orthopaedic surgeons were finding his demands increasingly difficult to manage, as he demanded more analgesia, further surgery and a management plan that involved "doing something". He had told the orthopaedic registrar that "I will kill myself if nothing is done".

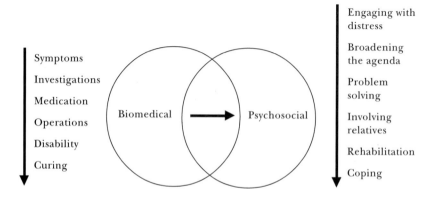

Fig. 8.1 *The shift from the biomedical to the psychosocial framework of care.*

He was reluctant to see a psychiatrist, but acknowledged that he had become desperate and disillusioned. The psychiatric registrar spoke with three other specialists involved in his care (infectious diseases, pain specialist and dermatologist), all of whom were finding his demands for a second opinion at a hospital outside the region difficult to manage.

After a discussion with his general practitioner, who knew the patient very well and confirmed that he had a history of extremely poor adaptation to disability in a previous illness, it was decided to hold a case conference at the pain clinic. All the relevant specialists were invited, as well as the general practitioner. It was agreed that there would be no further surgery or second opinion. A management plan would be implemented that was proactive and that involved helping him manage the pain, restricting his access to other specialists, providing support and generally helping him with pain-coping strategies. This plan would be implemented in the joint pain clinic with the psychiatrist and pain physician, with out-patient visits at monthly intervals. The plan was communicated to the general practitioner, who would also see him at regular intervals (every two months) and reinforce the management plan.

Opportunities for collaborative research

Joint service developments of the kind described often provide good opportunities for the discussion of collaborative research projects. The pain clinician, psychologist and psychiatrist, by combining their skills, may be better able to prepare and conduct research studies on pain patients than any single speciality alone. There are many successful precedents for such collaborative research endeavours (Pilowsky & Barrow, 1990; Williams *et al*, 1993).

Conclusions

The liaison psychiatrist has the opportunity to make an important contribution to the assessment and management of patients in pain clinics. It is important, however, for the liaison psychiatry service to be aware of the roles of other members of the multi-disciplinary pain team, which may include a psychologist, nurses, occupational therapists and physiotherapists. Whatever relationship is established with the local pain clinic, it is imperative to discuss the funding of the liaison psychiatry sessions. If this essential task is not undertaken, the liaison psychiatry service may become overwhelmed with referrals, which is likely to result in the service becoming inefficient and unpopular. Such an arrangement is clearly unsatisfactory, not only for the referrers, but also ultimately for the patients.

108   *Bass*

References

BARSKY, A. (1998) A comprehensive approach to the chronically somatizing patient. *Journal of Psychosomatic Research*, **45**, 301–306.

BASS, C. (1996) Management of somatisation disorder. *Prescribers' Journal*, **36**, 198–205.

BENJAMIN, S., BARNES, D., BERGER, S., *et al* (1988) The relationship of chronic pain, mental illness and organic disorders. *Pain*, **32**, 185–195.

——, MAWER, J. & LENNON, S. (1992) The knowledge and beliefs of family care givers about chronic pain patients. *Journal of Psychosomatic Research*, **36**, 211–217.

BOSTON, K., PEARCE, S. A. & RICHARDSON, P. H. (1990) The Pain Cognitions Questionnaire. *Journal of Psychosomatic Research*, **34**, 103–109.

CROFT, P., RIGBY, A. S., BOSWELL, R., *et al* (1993) The prevalence of chronic widespread pain in the general population. *Journal of Rheumatology*, **20**, 710–713.

DOLIN, S. J. & STEPHENS, J. (1998) Pain clinics and liaison psychiatry. *Anaesthesia*, **53**, 317–319.

DWORKIN, S. F., VON KORFF, M. & LE RESCHE, L. (1990) Multiple pains and psychiatric disturbance. *Archives of General Psychiatry*, **47**, 239–244.

FISHBAIN, D. A., GOLDBERG, M., MEAGHER, B. R., *et al* (1986) Male and female chronic pain patients categorised by DSM–III psychiatric diagnostic criteria. *Pain*, **26**, 181–197.

——, ——, Steele, R., *et al* (1991) Completed suicide in chronic pain. *Clinical Journal of Pain*, **7**, 29–36.

GILL, D. & BASS, C. (1997) Somatoform and dissociative disorders: assessment and treatment. *Advances in Psychiatric Treatment*, **3**, 9–16.

GOLDBERG, D., GASK, L. & O'DOWD, T. (1989) Teaching techniques of reattribution. *Journal of Psychosomatic Research*, **33**, 697–703.

GUTHRIE, E., CREED, F., DAWSON, D., *et al* (1991) A controlled trial of psychological treatment for irritable bowel syndrome. *Gastroenterology*, **100**, 450–457.

HARRIS, C. & BARRACLOUGH, B. M. (1994) Suicide as an outcome for medical disorders. *Medicine*, **73**, 281–296.

HOTOPF, M. (1998) Occupational factors and unexplained physical symptoms. *Advances in Psychiatric Treatment*, **4**, 151–158.

HOUSE, A. (1995) The patient with medically unexplained symptoms: making the initial psychiatric contact. In *Treatment of Functional Somatic Symptoms* (eds R. A. Mayou, C. Bass & M. Sharpe), pp. 89–102. Oxford: Oxford University Press.

JENSEN, M. P., KAROLY, P. & HUGER, R. (1987) The development and preliminary validation of an instrument to assess a patient's attitudes towards pain. *Journal of Psychosomatic Research*, **31**, 393–400.

KATON, W., EGAN, K. & MILLER, D. (1985) Chronic pain: lifetime psychiatric diagnoses and family history. *American Journal of Psychiatry*, **142**, 1156–1160.

KOUYANOU, K., PITHER, C. & WESSELY, S. (1997a) Medication misuse, abuse and dependence in chronic pain patients. *Journal of Psychosomatic Research*, **43**, 497–504.

——, —— & —— (1997b) Iatrogenic factors and chronic pain. *Psychosomatic Medicine*, **59**, 597–604.

MCQUAY, H. & MOORE, R. (1997) Antidepressants and chronic pain. *British Medical Journal*, **314**, 763–764.

PHELAN, M., WYKES, T. & GOLDMAN, H. (1994). Global functioning scales: a review. *Social Psychiatry and Psychiatric Epidemiology*, **29**, 205–211.

PILOWSKY, I. (1967) Dimensions of hypochondriasis. *British Journal of Psychiatry*, **113**, 89–93.

—— & BARROW, C. G. (1990) A controlled study of psychotherapy and amitriptyline used individually and in combination in the treatment of chronic, intractable "psychogenic" pain. *Pain*, **40**, 3–19.

ROSENSTIEL, A. K. & KEEFE, F. J. (1983) The use of cognitive coping strategies in chronic low back pain patients: relationships to patient characteristics and current adjustment. *Pain*, **17**, 33–44.

SHARPE, M. (1995) Cognitive behavioural therapies in the treatment of functional somatic symptoms. In *Treatment of Functional Somatic Symptoms* (eds R. A. Mayou, C. Bass & M. Sharpe), pp. 122–143. Oxford: Oxford University Press.

——, MAYOU, R., SEAGROATT, V., *et al* (1994) Why do doctors find some patients difficult to help? *Quarterly Journal of Medicine*, **87**, 187–193.

SKEVINGTON, S. M. (1995) *Psychology of Pain*. Chichester: Wiley.

SULLIVAN, M., TURNER, J. & ROMANO, J. (1991) Chronic pain in primary care. *Journal of Family Practice*, **32**, 193–199.

SWARTZMAN, L. C., GWADRY, F. G., SHAPIRO, A. P., *et al* (1994) The factor structure of the Coping Strategies Questionnaire. *Pain*, **57**, 311–316.

TURK, D. C. & OKIFUJI, A. (1999) Assessment of patients' reporting of pain: an integrated perspective. *Lancet*, **353**, 1784–1788.

WARE, J. E. & SHERBOURNE, C. D. (1992) A 36-item short form health survey (SF–36): results from the Medical Outcomes Study. *Medical Care*, **30**, 473–483.

WEINMAN, J., PETRIE, K., MOSS-MORRIS, R., *et al* (1996) The Illness Perception Questionnaire: a new method for assessing the cognitive representation of illness. *Psychology and Health*, **11**, 431–445.

WILLIAMS, A. C., NICHOLS, M. K., RICHARDSON, P. H., *et al* (1993) Evaluation of a cognitive behavioural programme for rehabilitating patients with chronic pain. *British Journal of General Practice*, **43**, 513–518.

ZIGMOND, A. A. & SNAITH, R. P. (1983) The Hospital Anxiety and Depression Scale. *Acta Psychiatrica Scandinavica*, **67**, 361–370.

9   Liaison psychiatry in the intensive care unit

JULIA GLEDHILL and GEOFFREY LLOYD

Over recent decades the intensive care unit (ICU) has become an established facility in most general hospitals. To the unfamiliar visitor it may appear as a mass of machines and monitors, with alarms unpredictably triggered. Screens continuously flash essential information to staff trained to interpret them. Drips and tubes are carefully located.

The patient lies at the centre of this technological complexity. Whatever serious illness or injury has necessitated admission to the ICU, it is important to remember that the ways in which patients react to this environment will be influenced by their own unique personality traits and mechanisms for coping with stress.

To medical professionals who do not work regularly as part of the ICU team, the unit may seem mysterious and confusing. In contrast to other general hospital wards, where the doors are open to consulting professionals and visitors, the doors to the ICU are routinely closed. Often it is necessary to ring a bell in order to gain admission.

In the UK, the liaison psychiatrist is not routinely a part of the team inside the doors and, in line with much liaison psychiatry practice, involvement in the work of the ICU at present is likely to take the form of patient consultations in response to specific requests. However, we believe liaison psychiatry has a far greater role to play in the work of the ICU and illustrate this in this chapter. At present such functions are incompletely recognised and resourced in the UK.

As do all people who are seriously ill, patients on an ICU utilise various psychological mechanisms in order to enable them to cope with the admission. At times this may lead to reactions which may be difficult for the attending staff to understand and this in turn may lead them to respond in a manner which is counter-therapeutic (often initiated at an unconscious level). This may cause difficulties in maintaining a working relationship between patient and staff and can result in problems with patient compliance. Some patients in ICUs go on to develop a formal psychiatric disorder.

Units which employ liaison psychiatrists as part of their staff have found them to be of great benefit in assisting with both the assessment and the management of individual patients and in promoting understanding among the staff of the dynamics within the unit, which in turn facilitates patient care (Billig, 1982).

In this chapter we first consider specific psychiatric disorders to which patients on an ICU may be particularly prone and how the liaison psychiatrist can help with assessment and management. Ways in which the psychiatrist can work with both the patient's relatives and the unit's staff are also discussed. We then outline the continuing role of the liaison psychiatrist after the discharge of patients from the unit. After a brief look at where liaison psychiatrists should work in this capacity, and how the service should be resourced, the chapter concludes by examining how such a service may be planned.

Disorders arising during ICU admission

The acutely behaviourally disturbed patient

For some time an entity known as the ICU syndrome (Kornfeld, 1971) was used to describe any gross behavioural or emotional disturbances occurring in the ICU, notably those with a psychotic element. Its aetiology was thought to be related to specific characteristics of the ICU environment. Sleep deprivation, constant noise, sensory monotony, the presence of monitoring equipment and the lack of orientating cues have all been implicated (Lloyd, 1993). These observations prompted changes in the design of ICUs and the ways in which the work of its staff was carried out. Efforts were made to reduce noise and to provide external windows and orientating cues such as clocks and calendars. The importance of sleep with a normal day–night cycle was acknowledged, as was the need for increased contact with attending staff and family members.

While the role of the ICU environment itself in causing psychological disturbance has been questioned (Holland *et al*, 1973) it is likely that it may contribute to the time of onset and maintenance of abnormalities in mental state. However, to attribute behavioural disturbance solely to the ICU environment is hazardous, as it minimises the need for a thorough assessment and diagnostic formulation. It also detracts from the very important distinction which needs to be made between delirium and an acute functional psychosis.

Delirium

Delirium always has an organic cause. According to ICD–10 (World Health Organization, 1992), it is characterised by concurrent disturbances of attention, perception, thinking, memory, psychomotor behaviour, emotion and the sleep–wake cycle, together with an impairment in the level of consciousness. Patients on ICUs are especially prone to such disorder because of the severe metabolic disturbances which may accompany their underlying physical disease process. Delirium is associated with a high mortality rate (Van Hemert *et al*, 1994), reflecting the seriousness of the underlying physical pathology. Prompt recognition is therefore essential if optimal treatment is to be instituted.

In the ICU, where admission is usually urgent and patients may be admitted unconscious, with little available history, aetiologies such as acute alcohol or drug withdrawal need to be considered when delirium presents within 72 hours of admission to hospital (alcohol) or up to six days (benzodiazepines).

An agitated patient often creates considerable anxiety for those around. This may be particularly so in the ICU, where attending staff are accustomed to nursing ventilated and sedated patients and the risk of detachment from essential supportive and monitoring equipment may be raised by behavioural disturbance. General advice to staff about optimising orientating cues and talking to patients in clear and simple terms, together with an explanation to staff that the symptoms are likely to resolve in time, may afford them great relief.

Advice on pharmacological treatments to reduce excessive agitation and to facilitate optimal patient care may also be helpful. Neuroleptics are most useful in this respect because of their calming effect together with their antipsychotic action. We recommend the use of haloperidol in the ICU, as it has fewer anticholinergic and anti-adrenergic effects. Droperidol can be used as an alternative for intravenous use in extreme emergency, titrating the dose according to the clinical response. However, in the case of delirium tremens following alcohol withdrawal, a benzodiazepine is the drug of choice, the dose of which should be reduced gradually over 7–10 days. It is also important to ensure that any patient coming through the ICU with a history of alcohol dependence is given high-dose thiamine to prevent the development of the Wernicke–Korsakoff syndrome.

Functional psychosis

A small proportion of physically ill hospital in-patients develop an acute and transient psychotic disorder (ICD–10). Out of a consecutive sample of 100 patients referred to psychiatric services from the general wards, 10 fulfilled this diagnosis (Cutting, 1980). It is often characterised by a well formed delusional system involving the staff immediately concerned with the patient's treatment (Lloyd, 1991). It seems that the aetiological importance of the physical illness is that it causes disruption to the patient's familiar environment (Cutting, 1980). Sensory deprivation, which has been reported in ICU environments, is known to be a contributory factor. Such disorders can lead to difficulties in management because patients, feeling threatened by or distrustful of staff, are likely to act in accordance with these delusional beliefs and may attempt to detach themselves from essential equipment, make efforts to leave the ICU or behave aggressively towards staff whom they believe are trying to harm them.

The development of such a disorder in a previously compliant patient may be difficult for attending medical staff to understand and the seemingly sudden change in behaviour may provoke strong reactions in the staff themselves. It is therefore vital to discuss with the staff the likely diagnosis and to explain why it may have occurred.

Acute and transient psychotic disorders are not unique to the ICU and they are almost always of short duration and usually resolve when the patient is discharged to more familiar surroundings. While discharge home is unlikely to be feasible in the ICU context, it may be possible to transfer the patient to a less threatening general ward, which may lead to symptom resolution. If this is not possible, antipsychotic medication is likely to be necessary. Again, haloperidol may be the best choice, as it is unlikely to cause significant haemodynamic upset. If a more rapid sedative effect is needed because, for example, of dangerously aggressive behaviour, a short-acting benzodiazepine such as lorazepam may be used.

In addition to pharmacological methods, the patient's mental state may be helped by minimising monitoring equipment and observations, as far as the physical condition permits, and a clear explanation to the patient of all procedures.

Affective disorder

Transient mood disturbances, particularly anxiety and depression, are to be expected after admission to an ICU. However, concern may arise when such affective change is more prolonged or interferes with the patient's physical condition (e.g. anxiety may cause an unacceptable rise in blood pressure). Such symptoms may also disrupt the ability of patients to comply with treatment or slow their progress, thus leading to a prolongation in their length of stay on the ICU.

For example, a depressed patient may form the belief that he will not recover (despite objective improvement) and thus refuse to engage in chest physiotherapy, leading to a deterioration in his physical condition, reinforcing his belief and prolonging his stay on the unit.

The psychological origins of such changes in the patient's physical condition are unlikely to be clear to attending staff and this is compounded by the fact that, for many ICU patients, oral communication may not be possible. Intubation and the inability to communicate have been shown to be the most stressful aspects of a stay on the ICU (Pennock *et al*, 1994) and are thus likely to contribute to the aetiology of affective changes.

Time is needed to make a careful clinical assessment, which may require the use of written communication or word boards. In addition, the psychiatrist has an important role in establishing, by reference to case notes and by speaking to relatives, whether there is a history of affective disorder and whether the patient was receiving any pharmacological treatment before admission which may have been inadvertently stopped.

The majority of patients on an ICU will exhibit transient mood disturbances and some may fulfil the criteria for a diagnosis of an adjustment disorder (ICD–10). This is usually self-limiting. Symptoms are likely to include anxiety about the possibility of death and about the strange and complex environment in which the patients find themselves, where many vital bodily functions seem to rely on complex machinery.

Staff may be advised that, in order to help alleviate symptoms of anxiety, it is important to provide reassurance by means of frequent explanations to the patient of what is happening and of the purpose of equipment and investigations (Baxter, 1974). Medication may be useful in some cases and we would recommend the use of benzodiazepines.

A depressed mood is not uncommon among ICU patients and can often be viewed as part of an adjustment disorder. However, if such symptoms persist longer or are more severe than those seen in adjustment disorder, consideration needs to be given as to whether diagnostic criteria for a depressive episode are being fulfilled. Often such a disorder is unrecognised, as there is an acceptance that such symptoms are a natural response to the patient's circumstances (Bronheim *et al*, 1985). The skills of a liaison psychiatrist are important in establishing the diagnosis and advising on treatment.

Supportive psychotherapy is helpful. It is important to acknowledge that depressive symptoms may be precipitated by the helplessness that many patients feel as a result of losing control over most of their bodily functions. Efforts to enable them to regain some influence over their situation may help. Careful thought needs to be given as to whether an antidepressant should be prescribed, as side-effects are likely to be poorly tolerated in the physically ill and benefits not seen for at least a week.

Tricyclic antidepressants may be more problematic in the physically ill and are often inadvisable in this group because of the possibility of serious cardiovascular side-effects. Selective serotonin reuptake inhibitors may be better tolerated in this group of patients, although the need for appropriate dose reduction in those with hepatic impairment must be remembered. Where an antidepressant is indicated, the possible risks need to be balanced against the likely benefits in each individual case and the liaison psychiatrist should continue to monitor the patient's mental state and response to medication. Clinical teams should be advised to continue anti-depressant treatment for at least six months after the resolution of symptoms.

The liaison psychiatrist can also help staff to make sense of their own reactions in response to their patient's affective state; for example, psychomotor retardation in the context of a depressive illness could be interpreted by staff as a deliberate unwillingness to cooperate with treatment, which may lead to feelings of irritation and anger and thus interfere with patient care. An understanding of the origins of such responses may help to facilitate the relationship between staff and patient.

Post-traumatic stress disorder

Over recent years, post-traumatic stress disorder (PTSD) has become increasingly recognised as a sequel to an event perceived by an individual as exceptionally threatening. It is therefore understandable that this syndrome is recognised in groups of patients admitted to ICUs. Among those admitted following road traffic accidents, for example, there is a 10% prevalence (Mayou *et al*, 1993) and among those admitted with severe burns there is a 7% prevalence at the time of discharge and more than 22% at four-month follow-up (Roca *et al*, 1992). It has also been noted in patients after myocardial infarction and coronary artery bypass surgery (Doerfler *et al*, 1994).

However, there are likely to be aspects of the patient's mode of admission to an ICU or experience on the unit which are themselves related aetiologically to symptoms of PTSD. These may include the seemingly sudden onset of life-threatening illness, necessitating ICU admission, which may be accompanied by feelings of intense fear, helplessness, a sense of loss of control and fears of death

(Doerfler *et al*, 1994). In addition, the rapidity with which investigations and treatments are carried out on the unit when the patient does not understand what is happening may perpetuate feelings of threat. Symptoms of PTSD are observed in a substantial proportion of patients who have endured traumatic illnesses or procedures in hospital (Williams *et al*, 1994). In addition, it is suggested that the likelihood of an individual developing this disorder is related to antecedent psychosocial problems (Mayou *et al*, 1993), the perceived extent of social support around the time of the trauma, and the degree of emotional distress and perceived helplessness, rather than a purely objective assessment of the severity of injury (Perry *et al*, 1992).

The psychiatrist on the ICU may have a useful role in trying to prevent or reduce such symptoms by advising the unit's staff about the importance of clear and frequent explanations and encouraging patients to verbalise their experiences early on. Some staff may feel wary of encouraging such discussion because of a fear of upsetting the patient.

Psychiatric assessment will be important in formulating a diagnosis and advising on treatment. Pharmacological treatments may be appropriate, such as benzodiazepines to reduce anxiety and facilitate sleep. Antidepressants may be helpful but the likely risks and benefits in the context of the underlying physical problems must be carefully evaluated. Psychological treatments, including behavioural therapy using graded exposure, cognitive techniques and psychodynamic therapy, may also be helpful (Solomon *et al*, 1992).

Post-traumatic stress disorder may be more prevalent in association with ICU admissions than is recognised, both because it is often currently not detected on the ICU and because symptoms may develop after discharge from hospital and follow-up may be undertaken by clinical teams from different disciplines not alert to this diagnosis. It has been suggested that patients could be screened for symptoms using rapidly administered instruments such as the Impact of Event Scale (Perry *et al*, 1992). However, the liaison psychiatrist may usefully contribute to the assessment of patients after discharge, which will facilitate the detection of such symptoms and determine the extent to which they are affecting the individual.

Mental health problems as a cause of ICU admission

These patients are usually admitted after episodes of deliberate self-harm. The group includes those who have taken overdoses sufficient to cause severe metabolic derangement, respiratory depression requiring mechanical ventilation, or organ failure. It also includes individuals with extensive injuries following self-inflicted burns, jumping from a height or under a moving vehicle and asphyxia by hanging. These patients are likely to have serious suicidal intent and a major psychiatric disorder, in contrast to patients who take drug overdoses, for whom there is no close correlation between the medical severity of the overdose and the seriousness of suicidal intent.

A psychiatric assessment is mandatory for all such patients during their hospital stay and it is useful for the ICU team to make the referral early. Although the patient may be unconscious at this stage, important information can be obtained from family and friends, and support can be provided for relatives. Evidence of persistent suicidal intent or a serious episode of self-harm in the context of a major psychiatric disorder is likely to lead to psychiatric admission once the patient has made a sufficient physical recovery. Patients who talk of discharging themselves may cause considerable anxiety for staff. It is important for the liaison psychiatrist to respond rapidly and sensitively to such concerns. For patients not agreeable to staying in hospital who are considered to be at risk of further self-harm or whose psychiatric disorder needs in-patient management, the Mental Health Act may need to be applied (see Chapter 6).

It is important that attending ICU staff are fully aware of the outcome of a psychiatric assessment and the proposed treatment plan. They can play a useful part in monitoring the individual's mental state.

Certain staff may have difficulty in accepting self-inflicted illness as a legitimate need for ICU resources and the psychiatrist can help staff to understand their feelings, which, if left unattended, may lead to responses such as anger, resentment and rejection, which may have a deleterious effect on patient care.

Pre-existing psychiatric disorder on the ICU

Patients with a history of psychiatric disorder may be admitted to the unit. Staff often seek advice about the use of psychotropic medication (Billig, 1982); if consistent and regular psychiatric liaison consultation is available, such aspects of the patient's care are likely to be attended to appropriately.

Working with relatives

The onset of life-threatening illness will have emotional repercussions for the immediate family of the ICU patient, and the ways in which they cope will influence the patient's outcome. The daily routine of certain families will for some time revolve around visits to the ICU and they will become familiar figures to the staff. For some, coming to terms with the severity of their relative's condition may be difficult and some may respond by denying what has happened. Anxiety may be high and this can be transmitted to patients, increasing their own anxiety and interfering with progress.

Family members often seek frequent reassurance about their relative's condition, particularly from the nursing staff who are readily available and have become familiar to them. This may lead to a difficult internal conflict for staff, between a wish to protect the family from upset on the one hand and a knowledge of the reality of the patient's physical condition on the other. The liaison psychiatrist can assist by discussing with staff the difficulties they may have in containing the emotional responses of family members, engaging in supportive work with relatives and, on occasion, facilitating discussions between staff and relatives.

Working with staff

Nursing staff form the most stable professional group on the ICU and the stresses and psychological difficulties of working in this environment have been recognised. Higher levels of depression, hostility and anxiety have been reported in this group than among those working in a non-ICU setting (Gentry *et al*, 1972). However, few units in the UK currently address these issues in a formal way.

The exposure of staff to the constant threat of death, combined with the hopes of patients and their families vested in their expertise, can at times lead to a sense of omnipotence but on other occasions may lead to feelings of helplessness and uselessness when treatment is unsuccessful. There are various ways in which the liaison psychiatrist can work with staff to help them to understand the emotional responses of their patients and to enable staff to acknowledge their own feelings. It is important to include teaching sessions on the psychological reactions of patients and staff to critical illness among the respective programmes for all ICU staff in training. In addition, if psychiatrists work on a unit where attendance at ward rounds or case reviews is an accepted role, they can assist in alerting staff to a patient's psychological difficulties or potential distress (Billig, 1982), which may be too painful for staff to acknowledge consciously. It is also important to remind staff of the need to talk to patients on ventilators and to allow patients to communicate their feelings (Billig, 1982).

When working in a consultative role it is important to talk initially with the attending staff about their observations regarding difficulties patients may be experiencing. It is also vital to feed back to staff the impression formed after a psychiatric assessment. The limitations of working purely in this way are that if staff are not familiar with the psychiatrist, who is then not viewed as an integral member of the ICU team, it may be hard for them to feel safe enough to volunteer difficulties that they may be encountering in caring for a particular patient. Interventions are therefore limited to a more general discussion of ways in which staff may be able to help their patient.

If, by attending the ICU daily and becoming a familiar figure to the staff, the liaison psychiatrist is seen as a member of the ICU team, the work that can be done with staff is likely to be more far-reaching. With this in mind, some ICUs have tried to utilise staff support groups. The varied success of this is likely to relate to how willing the staff are to explore the interpersonal dynamics within the ICU. The introduction of such an approach may be the beginning of an evolving process, which changes from an initial stage of formal acceptance and structure and develops over time as trust and confidence builds, such that meetings can become more free and open, with more widespread participation (Simon & Whiteley, 1977).

It is clear that different patients will evoke different emotional responses in attending staff (e.g. over-identification with a patient who shares several personal characteristics) and that such reactions will have an effect on the relationship between patient and staff members. For example, feelings of helplessness engendered by 'over-demanding' patients whose requests cannot be adequately met might be understood as a projection by the patients of their own powerlessness and lack of control. The provision of help in understanding such interactions may help staff members to work therapeutically with such patients.

The continuing role of the liaison psychiatrist after ICU discharge

In the same way that admission to an ICU can lead to a variety of emotional responses, discharge may also lead to psychological difficulties, both immediately and in the longer term.

Problems which arise during hospital admission are more likely to be noted than those beginning after discharge. While the ICU environment itself may lead to difficulties, the transition from the security of intensive monitoring, close observation and one-to-one nursing to the less intensive care on a general hospital ward may precipitate anxiety in some patients as well as in their close relatives

(Kiely, 1974). It has been observed that such responses on transfer out of the coronary care unit may be accompanied by cardiovascular complications such as arrhythmia and re-infarction, with an associated rise in catecholamine levels (Klein *et al*, 1968).

It is important to provide time for the discussion of plans for transfer from the ICU and to allow patients to explore their feelings about this. More specific interventions may include a transition from ICU to the general ward, with a graded reduction in the level of monitoring and support, together with cognitive–behavioural approaches to try to re-establish a sense of control within the patient and thus facilitate active care-taking on the part of the patient (Kiely, 1974).

We believe the liaison psychiatrist should continue to monitor the mental state of patients after discharge from the ICU and educate the general ward staff to try to ensure that patients have an opportunity to talk about some of the anxiety-provoking experiences they might have encountered in connection with their admission to hospital and to discuss any concerns they might have about their discharge home (Kornfeld, 1971).

Further psychological disorder may develop after hospital discharge. Because specific ICU follow-up clinics are rare and patients' homes may be geographically distant, such difficulties may remain undetected. General practitioners need to be aware of the possibility that psychological symptoms may develop many months after discharge. The presence of symptoms such as anxiety, PTSD and phobic anxiety, as well as being distressing for patients and their relatives, is likely to impair rehabilitation.

Where should the ICU liaison psychiatrist work?

It is unlikely that patients on the ICU will be able to move from their bed area for assessment. However, the need for confidentiality and privacy must not be forgotten. If possible, and with the agreement of the patient and the unit's staff, interviews can take place in the bed area with the curtains drawn.

It is important when consulting with the unit's staff not to discuss inappropriate matters around the patient's bed, even if the patient appears to be unconscious or heavily sedated. It is preferable to have this discussion in the privacy of an office or interview room on the unit. Segments of perceived conversation may be inappropriately interpreted by patients and this could worsen their affective state. Equally, if patients know their case is being discussed while they are excluded, paranoid feelings may be fuelled.

Staff support consultations should take place on the ICU, in an appropriately sized interview room if available, and a regular time should be fixed for this meeting each week. This will help to ensure that as many staff as possible attend. The ICU liaison psychiatrist has a valuable contribution to make to the day-to-day life of the unit. In helping to build a role as part of the ICU team, attendance at daily ward rounds is important. This may be a suitable forum for questions regarding psychotropic medication. It may also present an opportunity for a brief assessment of the patients' emotional wellbeing and to observe the dynamics between staff and patients and between staff members.

Why resource liaison psychiatry on the ICU?

We are unaware of any prospective systematic studies describing the total prevalence of psychiatric disorder in association with ICU admission. It is therefore difficult to quantify precisely such problems and there is clearly a need for prospective research in this area. However, cross-sectional surveys, most often based on coronary care units or looking at patients who have had cardiac surgery, have estimated that psychiatric difficulties complicate the care of 30–70% of patients in ICUs (Hackett *et al*, 1968). It is also recognised that rates of psychiatric disorder among patients with severe physical illness are at least twice those of the general population (House & Hodgson, 1994). In addition, many psychological disorders are unrecognised in the general hospital setting (Royal Colleges of Physicians and Psychiatrists Working Party, 1995). With these facts in mind, it seems likely that the need for a liaison psychiatry service in the ICU setting is considerable.

Without such a service, it is likely that overt behavioural changes signifying underlying psychological distress may go unrecognised by the ICU staff. The appropriate identification and treatment of psychological and psychiatric disorders are important. Their presence, as well as being extremely distressing for patients, is likely to retard their progress. Successful psychiatric intervention is likely to reduce mortality and morbidity rates, unnecessary investigations, length of stay and hospitalisation costs (House & Hodgson, 1994).

Planning the service

There are no national policies regarding the role of liaison psychiatry services on ICUs. For most UK hospitals, the position of the liaison psychiatrist on the unit is not clearly delineated and requests for psychiatric consultation are likely to be precipitated by acute difficulties. With these considerations in mind, it is important that regular dialogue is established between the clinicians and managers in charge of the ICU and the consultant liaison psychiatrist in order to consider the functions of such a service. While we do not believe that ICUs require the full-time attachment of a member of the liaison psychiatry team, we do suggest that consistent contact is established, such as by regular attendance at ward rounds, teaching sessions and special meetings with the unit's staff. At minimum, a liaison psychiatrist with access to a clinical psychologist could provide this. In addition to this, liaison consultation should be easily and rapidly accessible.

The service should be targeted at all patients having an episode of ICU care. In some cases, involvement could start before an elective admission and continue after ICU discharge. The aims of such a service would be to prevent, identify and treat psychiatric disorder in this patient group and to provide teaching and support to the unit's staff, helping them to recognise psychological difficulties in their patients and to better understand their own responses to the potentially stressful environment in which they work. Requests for psychiatric assessment should be rapidly met and treatment should be promptly instituted and appropriately monitored, in order to reduce the length of ICU and hospital stay and reduce morbidity and mortality. Such outcomes are likely to benefit patients, staff and purchasers, who potentially stand to make significant financial savings.

Purchasers of acute medical services will need to ensure that a liaison psychiatry service is included as part of the provider unit. The cost of this service should be included within the medical directorate's budget.

The establishment of such a service has implications for training. Specialist registrars with posts in liaison psychiatry must be afforded the experience of working in specialised liaison settings, including ICUs. Similarly, other mental health professionals, such as psychiatric nurses and psychologists, must have supervised experience of work in this setting.

As with any clinical service, monitoring its effectiveness is important and we would advocate the use of medical audit in order to assess whether the goals of such a service are being achieved.

We believe that the liaison psychiatrist has an important contribution to make to the ICU. Systematic studies are needed in order to quantify the need more precisely and thus assist with resource allocation. However, the current paucity of liaison psychiatry posts in the UK means that some of the potential and valuable ways of working which we have discussed are unable to be put into practice at present.

It is our hope that in future years the doors of the ICU will be opened to liaison psychiatry and that we will be able to contribute more fully to the work of the unit. However, before this can happen there will need to be a considerable expansion of liaison psychiatry posts at consultant and specialist registrar level.

References

BAXTER, S. (1974) Psychological problems of intensive care. *British Journal of Hospital Medicine*, 11, 875–885.

BILLIG, N. (1982) Liaison psychiatry: a role on the medical intensive care unit. *International Journal of Psychiatry in Medicine*, 11, 379–387.

BRONHEIM, H. E., IBERTI, T. J., BENJAMIN, E., *et al* (1985) Depression in the intensive care unit. *Critical Care Medicine*, 13, 985–988.

CUTTING, J. (1980) Physical illness and psychosis. *British Journal of Psychiatry*, 136, 109–119.

DOERFLER, L. A., PBERT, L. & DECOSIMO, D. (1994) Symptoms of post traumatic stress disorder following myocardial infarction and coronary artery bypass surgery. *General Hospital Psychiatry*, 16, 193–199.

GENTRY, W. D., FOSTER, S. B. & FROEHLING, S. (1972) Psychologic response to situational stress in intensive and nonintensive nursing. *Heart and Lung*, 31, 793.

HACKETT, T. P., CASSEM, N. H. & WISHNIE, H. A. (1968) The coronary care unit – an appraisal of its psychologic hazards. *New England Journal of Medicine*, 279, 1365–1370.

HOLLAND, J., SGROI, S. M., MARWIT, S. J., *et al* (1973) The ICU syndrome: fact or fancy? *International Journal of Psychiatry in Medicine*, 4, 241–249.

HOUSE, A. & HODGSON, G. (1994) Estimating needs and meeting demands. In *Liaison Psychiatry: Defining Needs and Planning Services* (eds S. Benjamin, A. House & P. Jenkins), pp. 3–15. London: Gaskell.

KIELY, W. F. (1974) Psychiatric aspects of critical care. *Critical Care Medicine*, 2, 139–142.

KLEIN, R. F., KLINER, V. S., ZIPES, D. P., *et al* (1968) Transfer from a coronary care unit. *Archives of Internal Medicine*, 122, 104–108.

KORNFELD, D. S. (1971) Psychiatric problems of an intensive care unit. *Medical Clinics of North America*, 55, 1353–1363.

LLOYD, G. G. (1991) *Textbook of General Hospital Psychiatry*. Edinburgh: Churchill Livingstone.

—— (1993) Psychological problems and the intensive care unit, *British Medical Journal*, 307, 458–459.

MAYOU, R., BRYANT, B. & DUTHIE, R. (1993) Psychiatric consequences of road traffic accidents. *British Medical Journal*, 307, 647–651.

PENNOCK, B. E., CRASHAW, L., MAHER, T., *et al* (1994) Distressful events in the ICU as perceived by patients recovering from coronary artery bypass surgery. *Heart and Lung*, 23, 323–327.

PERRY, S., DIFEDE, J., MUSNGI, M., *et al* (1992) Predictors of post traumatic stress disorder after burn injury. *American Journal of Psychiatry*, 149, 931–935.

ROCA, R. P., SPENCE, R. J. & MUNSTER, A. M. (1992). Post traumatic adaptation and distress among adult burn survivors. *American Journal of Psychiatry*, 149, 1234–1238.

ROYAL COLLEGES OF PHYSICIANS AND PSYCHIATRISTS WORKING PARTY (1995) *The Psychological Care of Medical Patients*. London: Royal College of Physicians.

SIMON, N. M. & WHITELEY, S. (1977) Psychiatric consultation with MICU nurses: the consultation conference as a working group. *Heart and Lung*, **6**, 497–504.

SOLOMON, S. D., GERRITY, E. T. & MUFF, A. M. (1992) Efficacy of treatments for post traumatic stress disorder. *Journal of the American Medical Association*, **268**, 633–638.

VAN HEMERT, A. M., VAN DER MAST, R. C., HENGEVELD, M. W., *et al* (1994) Excess mortality in general hospital patients with delirium: a 5-year follow-up of 519 patients seen in psychiatric consultation. *Journal of Psychosomatic Research*, **38**, 339–346.

WILLIAMS, S. L., WEIR, L. & WALDMANN, C. (1994) Post traumatic stress disorder in the ICU setting. *Care of the Critically Ill*, **10**, 77–79.

WORLD HEALTH ORGANIZATION (1992) *The ICD–10 Classification of Mental and Behavioural Disorders*. Geneva: WHO.

10 Mental health services for people with HIV/AIDS

JOSE CATALAN and TREVOR FRIEDMAN

Infection with HIV continues to be a siginificant problem in the UK: by the end of 1998 nearly 30 000 people were estimated to be living with the infection, about one-third undiagnosed (Communicable Disease Report, 1999*a*). The number of adults living with diagnosed HIV infection in England, Wales and Northern Ireland rose by 29% between the end of 1995 (14 200) and the end of 1998 (18 300). During this period, infections acquired as a result of heterosexual exposure increased by 72%, those due to sex between men by 23% and those due to injecting drugs of misuse by 3% (Communicable Disease Report, 1999*b*). Increase in the prevalence of HIV infection is likely to be the result of both a reduction in mortality due to the introduction of new and effective treatments, and the continued spread of the infection, with new cases occurring regularly. Although a slowing down in the rate of spread of the infection was expected, current figures are starting to exceed predictions made in recent years (Day Report, 1996). Preliminary figures from the Public Health Laboratory Service (PHLS) reported in January 2000 showed the largest ever number of new infections in 1999, with a total of 2457 new cases, 1070 resulting from heterosexual sex and 989 from sex between men (*Evening Standard*, 2000).

The majority of cases of HIV infection have been identified in London, the two Thames Regions accounting for almost 70% of AIDS cases, a pattern which is expected to continue well into the new century. Geographically, the real picture may be slightly different: the place where a diagnosis of AIDS is made and thus from where reporting occurs is not co-terminus with the patient's area of residence. It is quite possible that psychiatric or other health problems will sometimes develop away from the south-east of England, where many AIDS cases have been reported and patients may be receiving treatment. However, even with this qualification, it is clear that the number of patients and hence the pattern of needs and services will vary considerably between the large metropolitan areas and the rest of the country (Catalan, 1997*a*).

Mental health needs of people with HIV infection

Individuals with HIV infection can experience a range of mental disorders related to their need to adjust to a potentially fatal disorder and to central nervous involvement. While these disorders are comparable to those faced by other individuals with severe and disabling conditions, such as cancer, the stigma associated with HIV infection and the presence of a psychiatric history in a substantial proportion of people with HIV add to the risk of the development of psychiatric morbidity. A brief outline of the mental health problems seen in people with HIV infection is given here. More detailed information is available elsewhere (Catalan *et al*, 1995; Rabkin, 1996; Catalan, 1997*b*, 1999).

Factors contributing to mental disorders in HIV infection

Most people with HIV infection experience some degree of psychological and social disturbance, although only a minority, possibly about a third of all patients, suffer more severe and sometimes persistent disorders.

The risk of developing substantial psychological morbidity is influenced by a variety of factors. Some are related to the HIV infection itself, such as those problems arising at the time of HIV diagnosis, or in association with severe physical symptoms or treatment side-effects, as tends to occur in advanced HIV disease. A psychiatric history or personality disorder and the absence of social supports are important predictors of psychological morbidity. A coping style characterised by avoidance, denial and use of non-active strategies, and exposure to adverse life events, including grief due to loss of friends to AIDS, are associated with poorer adjustment. Injecting drug users are more likely than other groups to experience problems, and this is of particular relevance in geographical areas where injecting drug users are the main HIV population, as is the case in parts of Scotland. In US studies, gender, age and ethnicity have been shown to contribute to the development of psychological morbidity (see Catalan *et al*, 1995 for review).

Factors contributing to referral to mental health services

Not all patients experiencing psychological problems are identified as such by the doctors and nurses providing general medical care, as has been shown in primary and secondary care. A variety of factors concerning the patients, type of psychiatric symptoms, training and skills of frontline medical and nursing staff, and the extent and availability of sources of mental health intervention, will affect the rates and patterns of referrals.

Patients with high expectations of care who wish to be actively involved in decisions about their treatment may well verbalise their needs and problems more clearly than those more prone to accept doctors' recommendations without question. The discovery of a psychiatric history may lead doctors to refer for further psychiatric care, even in the absence of clear psychiatric symptoms. Demanding patients, or those with a history of difficult behaviour or violence, sometimes lead medical staff to reach for help from mental health workers.

Severe and dramatic symptoms or signs of mental illness or distress, such as suicidal ideas or acts and disturbed or aggressive behaviour, are more likely to lead to referral than less overt evidence of distress. Misunderstandings between patients and doctors about management may sometimes lead to referral to mental health services when doctors believe that "patients must be ill if they cannot appreciate what we are trying to do to help".

The experience and training of frontline staff will affect the likelihood of their asking the right questions to elicit symptoms of mental disorder, as will their confidence and skills in dealing with distress, suicidal ideas or unhappiness.

Ease of access to mental health services will lead not only to more referrals, but also to a larger proportion of less severe disorders being seen by the specialist team. While this may be desirable, as it could lead to early intervention and thus the prevention of either deterioration or the development of more severe problems, there is a danger of the service being swamped by minor problems which are self-limiting and do not require specialist involvement.

The presence of competent and experienced health advisers and social workers will ensure that the less severe problems are dealt with by non-specialists, provided they have access to the mental health team for discussion and referral. Local voluntary and independent support services may also support people in psychological and social distress.

Types of mental disorders in HIV infection

In general, psychiatric syndromes among people infected with HIV have been found to have a higher prevalence than in the general population, and one that is comparable to that found in other people with significant physical disorders. A number of studies have shown that individuals who regard themselves as at risk of infection, seek HIV testing and are found to be negative have comparable levels of current psychological morbidity and lifetime prevalence of psychiatric disorders to people who are HIV positive. This finding has implications for the provision of mental health backup in genitourinary medicine (GUM) departments and other facilities where HIV testing is carried out.

Abnormal psychological reactions

Adjustment disorder is the most common diagnosis among people referred to mental health services (up to 30%); it is often characterised by depressive symptoms and behavioural problems, sometimes including substance misuse. Personality disorders are often associated with it.

Affective disorders and syndromes

Major depression has been reported in up to 8% of people with HIV infection, and some reports have found elevated rates of dysthymia. The risk of manic disorders is increased in people with advanced and symptomatic HIV infection, and is often associated with cognitive impairment. Manic patients usually require admission to a psychiatric ward. Suicidal behaviour is not uncommon, many reports showing an increased rate of completed suicide 7–36 times that of sex- and age-matched controls. Persistent anxiety disorders are present in about 5% of people with HIV infection, while brief episodes of anxiety are common.

Organic brain syndromes

Acute and chronic brain syndromes can occur in HIV, sometimes due to cerebral complications such as secondary infections and tumours, or as a result of primary HIV effects. HIV-associated dementia develops in up to 10% of people with AIDS, usually in the last year of life. Minor cognitive impairment is more common, possibly affecting up to one-third of AIDS patients. Secondary cerebral infections and tumours can affect up to about 20% of patients.

Abnormal beliefs in people seeking HIV testing

As mentioned above, psychological morbidity is high among those seeking testing, including those who are subsequently found to be uninfected. Some remain concerned about being infected even after repeated negative HIV tests. Beliefs and worries about infection in such cases should be regarded as a symptom, rather than a diagnosis, and further assessment needs to be performed to establish the cause (e.g. delusional disorder, hypochondriasis or obsessional disorder).

Mental disorders in partners and relatives

Partners and close family members will suffer variable levels of distress and psychological and social difficulties, in particular when dealing with severe health problems and in the terminal stages of care. The impact on children, whether infected or not, could be substantial, in particular when both parents are HIV positive (Sherr, 1991).

Referrals to liaison mental health services

To illustrate the pattern of referrals of HIV-related problems to liaison services, details are given here concerning a specialist service in central London, developed alongside the HIV/GUM service at the Chelsea and Westminster Hospital, where a quarter of the AIDS cases in the UK have been reported. The Psychological Medicine Unit was established in 1989, and it includes psychiatrists, psychologists and liaison psychiatric nurses. While the unit provides general mental health services to the general hospital and therefore receives referrals from all medical and surgical specialities, about 60% of its activity is concerned with HIV-related referrals.

In recent years there has been a substantial change in the nature of psychiatric problems referred to the service, reflecting the changing prognosis and morbidity of HIV infection following the introduction of the new anti-retroviral treatments in 1996. To illustrate this change, the diagnosis given to people with HIV newly referred to the Psychological Medicine Unit in 1990, 1995 and 1999 are discussed below.

As Table 10.1 shows, there has been a substantial increase in new referrals by comparison with the 1990 figures, 1995 showing an increase of 149% and 1999 193%. However, the number of people with HIV cared for at the Chelsea and Westminster Hospital during this period remained stable, at about 2200 patients per year.

TABLE 10.1

Principal psychiatric diagnosis of HIV patients referred to the Psychological Medicine Unit at Chelsea and Westminster Hospital, London, by year

Diagnosis	1990 n=123 (%)	1995 n=306 (%)	1999 n=360 (%)
Depression[1]	21 (17)	59 (19)	98 (27)
Anxiety disorder[2]	6 (5)	35 (11)	48 (13)
Adjustment disorder	33 (27)	25 (8)	44 (12)
Sexual dysfunction	1 (1)	5 (2)	46 (13)
Substance misuse[3]	21 (17)	22 (7)	32 (9)
Organic brain disorder	16 (13)	23 (8)	20 (6)
acute	5 (4)	5 (2)	14 (4)
chronic	11 (9)	18 (6)	6 (2)
Mania	4 (3)	7 (2)	0 (0)
Schizophrenia	1 (1)	2 (1)	4 (1)
No diagnosis	4 (3)	105 (34)	48 (13)

1. Includes major depression and dysthymia.
2. Includes anxiety, panic disorder, phobias and obsessive–compulsive disorder.
3. Includes alcohol and drug misuse.

The principal psychiatric diagnoses given to patients illustrate some of the changes mentioned. Thus, the proportion of depressive disorders almost doubled between 1990 and 1999, those in the latter year representing almost one-third of all diagnoses. By contrast, adjustment disorders showed the opposite pattern, from being the most common diagnosis in 1990 to being the fourth most common in 1990. Anxiety disorders also increased in frequency during the survey period.

The most dramatic change is seen in the increase in patients presenting with sexual dysfunction. While sexual problems were known to be common in HIV infection before new HIV treatments were developed, the reduction in morbidity and general improvements in quality of life resulting from the anti-retroviral treatments have led many patients to wish to return to a normal emotional and sexual life, seeking help for erectile dysfunction and related problems. Attention given by the media to new treatments for sexual dysfunction may also have contributed to the increased demand for help.

While these figures give some idea of the nature of the mental health problems faced by individuals with HIV infection, it is important to note that the content of their concerns and the nature of the problems experienced have also changed. Concerns about death and survival or the reactions of others to the infection have been replaced by the difficulties of adjusting to an unexpecetd extension in life expectancy, uncertainty about the long-term benefits of treatment, the need to maintain a very high level of treatment adherence, and the difficulties involved in normalising sexual and emotional life (Catalan *et al*, 2000).

Meeting the mental health needs of people with HIV infection

The local prevalence of HIV infection and the size and extent of the medical services for its diagnosis and treatment will determine the extent of the mental health services required for this patient group. The degree to which existing mental health services, including liaison psychiatry, are able to meet these needs will obviously be influenced by local circumstances.

Nature of mental health services required

A liaison mental health service, including liaison psychiatry, health psychology and nursing, would meet the needs of this patient group. Consultation and liaison facilities are essential, although the actual organisation and extent of facilities will be determined by local circumstances. There is little evidence that psychiatric in-patient facilities specifically for people with HIV infection are required, as only a minority of individuals will need admission, and they could be accommodated within existing resources. People with HIV-associated dementia are sometimes in need of residential care, but this can usually be provided by a combination of general hospital, respite and hospice care, with additional home-based community support.

Mental health consultation

There is a need for both the urgent assessment of in-patients and less urgent out-patient assessment. In-patient referrals tend to include people suffering from disorders such as suicidal ideas, organic brain syndromes, psychotic disorders with behavioural manifestations and problems related to substance misuse. Out-patient assessment covers the whole range of problems indicated in Table 10.1.

The services of a psychiatrist are often needed by in-patients, as psychotropic medication may be required and decisions may have to be made about admission to a psychiatric facility. Psychiatric liaison nurses play an important role in the assessment of in-patients, sometimes being the first point of contact, and here the nurse is in a good position to screen the patient and take steps to refer to the appropriate team member.

Psychologists and psychiatrists are usually required to deal with the range of psychiatric disorders seen in out-patient referrals. Neuropsychological assessment by trained psychologists will be required to establish the presence of HIV-related cognitive impairment and dementia.

Mental health interventions

After assessment, a variety of interventions may be required: psychological, such as cognitive–behavioural therapy, crisis intervention and supportive therapy; psychopharmacological, for example antidepressants and major tranquillisers; and psychosocial, involving work with hospital and community teams to ensure that the necessary supports are in place.

In a number of cases, access to members of the mental health team over a long period of time will be needed: worsening health problems and social difficulties may recur and easy access to mental health services may prevent crisis. Decisions will need to be made in some cases about the appropriateness of involving generic psychiatric services in the care of particular patients, as opposed to restricting contact to the liaison mental health team. For example, patients with schizophrenic disorders or bipolar illnesses who happen to be HIV positive may be better managed by the generic psychiatric services.

Prevention of HIV spread can also be a target of mental health intervention; this may take the form of either general educational measures to minimise the risks associated with injecting drug use and sexual transmission, or more specific interventions aimed at individuals who experience difficulties maintaining safer sexual practices, in which case cognitive–behavioural approaches can be very effective.

Mental health liaison

Regular contact between the mental health team and others involved in the care of patients with HIV is desirable in a number of settings:

(a) *Medical and nursing teams.* The presence of members of the liaison psychiatry team at medical ward rounds, ward multi-disciplinary meetings and discharge meetings will help with the identification of the mental health needs of patients, provide support to staff dealing with complex problems, and facilitate the setting up of review meetings and case conferences.

(b) *HIV testing sites*. GUM departments, antenatal clinics and other settings where HIV testing is performed usually have well trained staff (health advisers, nurses, doctors) who are involved in providing pre- and post-test information and support. Access to mental health specialists for discussion of difficult problems, potential referrals or management advice is generally welcome.

(c) *General practitioners*. Until fairly recently, HIV care has tended to be hospital based, and the skills of general practitioners have not been fully utilised. Patients' fears about confidentiality or negative attitudes meant that general practitioners often were unaware of their patients' health problems. Many HIV treatment centres now have a deliberate policy of involving general practitioners in the care of patients, including the mental health aspects. Links with general practitioners and practice nurses can ensure that there is backup to deal with the complex needs of patients with cognitive impairment or families with one or more HIV-infected members.

(d) *Respite care and hospices*. As the disease progresses, the needs for physical and mental care tend to increase, and respite care or terminal care may be required. People with longstanding psychological difficulties may need greater mental health input at this stage, while other individuals may develop cognitive impairment or other problems requiring mental health assessment and treatment.

Organisation of services

In the early years of the AIDS epidemic, health funds were separately identified to deal with the problem, but this 'ring fencing' is now disappearing. In areas of high HIV prevalence or where the development of clinical services has attracted large numbers of patients, as has occurred in the south-east of England, mental health services were developed to deal with the needs of these patients. The pattern and extent of these mental health services have been varied, partly driven by local need but also by the degree of interest and enthusiasm of different mental health professional groups. Three patterns of mental health services for HIV seem to have developed.

First, in many areas with low prevalence of HIV infection, existing mental health services, including liaison psychiatry, have provided whatever care was needed. In most instances, severe psychiatric disorders would be identified and treated by the generic services without resort to any other separately funded specialists or facilities.

Second, in areas close to district general hospitals or universities, where a small but important group of HIV patients receive medical care, the pattern has been to create part-time or occasionally full-time posts to work with GUM departments or with the in-patient medical unit. Clinical psychologists have often been employed to work alongside doctors and health advisers. Consultant psychiatrist sessions have sometimes been established, but the development of mental health services has not tended to be part of a carefully worked out plan, but rather of a series of individual initiatives.

Third, in metropolitan areas with high HIV prevalence, mostly in London, more comprehensive services have developed, usually involving psychiatrists, psychologists and psychiatric nurses. The degree to which these professional groups work together in one unit or are part of separate organisations has varied between centres. Again, the extent to which these newly funded services work exclusively with HIV patients or whether they provide generic liaison mental health to the general hospital has not been consistent. In some centres, general hospital mental health facilities have been possible only as a result of the development of HIV mental health teams.

Changes in funding for HIV in future will make it harder to develop separate services, something which is probably desirable, as integration with general psychiatric and liaison services is likely to lead to better use of resources.

In line with the recommendations of a report by the Royal College of Physicians and Royal College of Psychiatrists (1995) on the psychological care of medical patients, team work by psychiatrists, psychologists and psychiatric nurses would be likely to provide the best model of assessment and care.

Acknowledgements

The authors are grateful to Jennifer Barraclough, Ian Everall, Brian Gazzard, Paul Jenkins, Christine McLeod, Rashmi Shukla and Anne Tait, who were involved in earlier discussion of some the issues covered in this chapter.

References

CATALAN, J. (1997*a*) Services in London for HIV/AIDS-related mental health needs. In *London's Mental Health – The Report of the King's Fund London Commission*. London: King's Fund Publishing.
—— (1997*b*) The psychiatry of HIV infection. *Advances in Psychiatric Treatment*, **3**, 17–24.

—— (ed.) (1999) *Mental Health and HIV Infection*. London: UCL Press.

——, BURGESS, A. P. & KLIMES, I. (1995) *Psychological Medicine of HIV Infection*. Oxford: Oxford University Press.

——, MEADOWS, J., & DOUZENIS, A. (2000) *The Changing Pattern of Mental Health Problems in HIV Infection: The View from London, UK*. London: AIDS Care (in press).

COMMUNICABLE DISEASE REPORT (1997) AIDS and HIV-1 infection in the United Kingdom: monthly report. *Communicable Disease Report*, **7** (4), 29–32.

COMMUNICABLE DISEASE REPORT (1999*a*) AIDS and HIV infection in the United Kingdom: monthly report. *Communicable Disease Report*, **9** (48), 431–433.

COMMUNICABLE DISEASE REPORT (1999*b*) Survey of diagnosed HIV infections shows prevalence is rising. *Communicable Disease Report*, **9** (47), 415.

DAY REPORT (1996) The incidence and prevalence of AIDS and prevalence of other severe HIV disease in England and Wales for 1995 to 1999: projections using data to the end of 1994. *Communicable Disease Report*, **1**, R1–R24.

EVENING STANDARD (2000) Fear of big rise in AIDS victims. 28 January.

RABKIN, J. (1996) Prevalence of psychiatric disorders in HIV illness. *International Review of Psychiatry*, **8**, 157–166.

ROYAL COLLEGE OF PHYSICIANS & ROYAL COLLEGE OF PSYCHIATRISTS (1995) *The Psychological Care of Medical Patients: Recognition of Need and Service Provision*. London: Royal College of Physicians and Royal College of Psychiatrists.

SHERR, L. (1991) *HIV and AIDS in Mothers and Babies*. Oxford: Blackwell Scientific.

11 Liaison psychiatry in the maternity hospital

MARGARET OATES

Maternity hospitals are but one part of an integrated maternity service which includes the general practitioner and community midwife and extends from the confirmation of pregnancy until the six-week postnatal check. The nature of the patients, the organisation of the services and the rates of psychiatric disorder associated with childbirth are all different from those found in general hospitals.

Distinctive features of obstetric liaison psychiatry

The majority of women will use maternity services two or three times in their lifetime. With a few exceptions, these women are not ill and the traditional relationships with doctors and nurses based upon the sick role will not be appropriate. In general, these well women will be happy and excited to be pregnant and will expect their experience of maternity care to be positive, pleasant and emotionally meaningful.

Pregnant and post-partum women have a number of pre-arranged and structured contacts with hospital services over a limited time. This offers a unique opportunity for the detection of mental ill health and intervention.

The majority of women will receive 'shared care', that is, they will be cared for by their general practitioners and hospital obstetricians, and by community and hospital midwives. Most will be delivered by a midwife and will leave hospital in the hours or days after delivery, their post-partum care being carried out at home. A liaison psychiatrist to an obstetric unit therefore has to relate as much to general practitioners and community midwives as to hospital-based staff.

Although it has been established that women are at greatly elevated risk of developing a serious affective disorder after delivery, the majority of these women will be well during pregnancy (Kendell *et al*,

1987; Cox *et al*, 1993). However, some may have risk factors which can be detected early in the pregnancy and this may enable the liaison psychiatrist to anticipate and even prevent such an illness (O'Hara & Swain, 1996). Despite the early onset of the most severe illnesses, most psychiatric illnesses will present after the woman has left hospital. The liaison psychiatrist to an obstetric unit therefore has to be able to continue managing patients after discharge.

Women who become ill will require a range of resources, including out-patient clinics, community psychiatric nurses and in-patient mother-and-baby beds. The obstetric liaison psychiatrist therefore needs to work with a multi-disciplinary perinatal psychiatry team. This team should work both in maternity hospitals and in the community (Oates, 1996).

Psychiatric morbidity associated with pregnancy and childbirth

Normal emotional changes following childbirth

Between 60% and 80% of women experience 'the blues', an essentially normal and self-limiting state of emotional turbulence, restlessness and insomnia, which occurs between the third and the tenth post-partum day. 'The blues' usually therefore occurs at home and is familiar to community midwives. Although forewarned, most women will be quite distressed and sometimes women in these states are referred to a psychiatrist. It is important for the liaison psychiatry team and the maternity staff to have an understanding of the full range of normal emotions, including distress, that follow childbirth. It may take between six and eight weeks for a woman to regain her normal emotional state. During this time, the woman's capacity to cope with stress may be lowered, particularly when tired. It is also common for first-time mothers to experience some anxiety with the establishment of breastfeeding, difficult babies and new routines.

Postnatal depression

It is estimated that approximately 10% of all women become sufficiently depressed to meet the Research Diagnostic Criteria (Cox *et al*, 1993) for major depression in the year after childbirth. Approximately 3–5% of all women delivered will suffer from a moderate to severe major depressive illness that requires treatment (Cox *et al*, 1993) and 1.7% of women will be referred to a psychiatrist with a new episode of psychiatric disorder (Oates, 1995). Some of the risk factors for major postnatal depression – most importantly a previous history of postnatal depression – can be identified in the antenatal period. These women should be identified and perhaps seen after delivery. In the case of very severe episodes, consideration may be given to prophylactic antidepressants.

For the more numerous, less severe forms of postnatal depressive illness, a number of psychosocial risk factors have been identified. This has led some workers to engage in innovative antenatal intervention programmes (Elliott, 1989). A liaison psychiatrist together with the other members of the liaison team and the maternity staff would be ideally placed to develop such intervention programmes. Frequent antenatal admission late in pregnancy for non-specific reasons may also indicate psychiatric problems and become a focus for intervention.

Puerperal psychosis

Approximately 2 per 1000 women delivered will need to be admitted to a psychiatric hospital suffering from a psychotic illness. The true incidence of puerperal psychosis is probably double this. These psychoses are very florid and usually present acutely between the fifth and sixteenth post-partum day (Kendell *et al*, 1987; Oates, 1996). They may present in maternity hospitals, but more commonly via community services. They frequently represent a psychiatric emergency and may require prompt admission to a mother-and-baby unit, although sometimes they can be managed at home.

Some women at high risk of developing a puerperal psychosis can be identified in the antenatal clinic. These will include those with a history of puerperal psychosis or a history of non-puerperal manic–depressive illness (the risk is 1 in 2 to 1 in 3) (Wieck *et al*, 1991). Although women with chronic schizophrenia are not at greatly elevated risk of a relapse after delivery, women with episodic paranoid schizophrenia may be at a risk equivalent to that of manic–depressive illness (Davies *et al*, 1995). The liaison psychiatrist will need to be aware of these patients antenatally and at least closely monitor them after delivery. Prophylaxis with a mood stabiliser or neuroleptic from the first post-partum day may substantially reduce the risk of such illness.

Pre-existing psychiatric disorder

Few psychiatric conditions, with the exception of eating disorders, are associated with a reduction in fertility. Women suffering from a range of psychiatric problems will therefore present during the antenatal period. Phobic anxiety states, panic disorder and obsessive–compulsive disorder may deteriorate during pregnancy and the post-partum period. They will require expert psychiatric management. Women with chronic schizophrenia and recurrent bipolar disorder may also become pregnant. They will require sophisticated, collaborative management on the part of the obstetrician and psychiatrist, and a careful balancing of the risks to the mother's mental health against the risks to the developing foetus of continuing psychotropic medication.

Antenatal psychiatric disorder

In contrast to the greatly elevated risk of psychiatric illness post-partum, pregnancy is not associated with an increased incidence of new psychiatric disorder. Despite this, minor depressive illness and generalised anxiety is common, particularly in the first trimester. Most of these conditions are self-limiting, and their prevalence drops sharply in the second and third trimesters; none the less, the liaison psychiatrist will receive referrals of distressed pregnant women.

Vulnerable groups

Disabling states of psychological distress will frequently occur in relation to a loss of pregnancy, the antenatal diagnosis of foetal abnormality, medically complicated pregnancies, premature deliveries, and babies in special-care baby units.

Estimating service resources required

An average health district serving a population of 350 000 with a maternity hospital delivering approximately 5000 babies a year can expect the per annum rates shown in Table 11.1. The referral rate to psychiatric services can be doubled if it includes women referred

TABLE 11.1
Average annual incidence of psychiatric referral from a maternity hospital delivering approximately 5000 babies a year

Cause of referral	No. of women	%
New episode of depressive illness	500	10
Moderate to severe major depressive illness	150–250	3–5
New episode of psychiatric disorder	125	1.7
Admission to a psychiatric hospital	20	
Puerperal psychosis requiring admission	10	

during the antenatal period and those referred with pre-existing psychiatric disorder (between 300 and 500 a year).

It can be seen that meeting the psychiatric needs of a recently delivered population, which includes the liaison service to a maternity hospital, requires, for a standard health district, between three and five sessions a week of a consultant psychiatrist's time. This can be adjusted according to the actual birth rate.

Functions of a liaison obstetric perinatal psychiatric team

The liaison services to a maternity hospital should be seen as part of a comprehensive perinatal psychiatry service, which will include not only specified specialist consultant sessions but also the services of a multi-disciplinary team, whose key members should be specialist community psychiatric nurses. The perinatal psychiatrist and team can therefore provide both general and liaison psychiatric services (Oates, 1996).

The main functions of the team would be as follows:

(a) to offer prenatal counselling to those women at high risk of developing a post-partum psychiatric disorder;
(b) to accept referrals from the antenatal clinic of high-risk women who are well;
(c) to see, offer advice to and manage, when appropriate, distressed pregnant women, particularly those from vulnerable subgroups;
(d) to assist in the management of mentally ill pregnant women and liaise with obstetricians and general adult psychiatrists;
(e) to plan postnatal psychiatric care and intervention for women at high risk;
(f) to provide a liaison consultation service to the postnatal wards;
(g) to manage significant psychiatric disorder arising in the puerperium in the community and out-patient clinics, and on an in-patient mother-and-baby unit;
(h) to make a contribution to the undergraduate and postgraduate education of general practitioners, obstetricians and midwives.

References

Cox, J. L., Murray, D. & Chapman, G. (1993) A controlled study of the onset prevalence and duration of postnatal depression. *British Journal of Psychiatry*, **163**, 27–31.

DAVIES, A., McIVOR, R. J. & KUMAR, C. (1995) Impact of childbirth on a series of schizophrenic mothers: a comment on the possible influence of oestrogen on schizophrenia. *Schizophrenia Research*, **16**, 25–31.

ELLIOTT, S. A. (1989) Psychological strategies in the prevention and treatment of postnatal depression. *Baillière's Clinical Obstetrics and Gynaecology*, **3**, 879–904.

KENDELL, R. F., CHALMERS, I. & PLATZ, C. (1987) The epidemiology of puerperal psychoses. *British Journal of Psychiatry*, **150**, 662–673.

OATES, M. R. (1995) Risk and childbearing. *Advances in Psychiatric Treatment*, **1**, 146–153.

—— (1996) Psychiatric services for women following childbirth. *International Review of Psychiatry*, **1**, 87–98.

O'HARA, M. W. & SWAIN, A. M. (1996) Rates and risk of post partum depression – a meta-analysis. *International Review of Psychiatry*, **1**, 87–98.

WIECK, A., KUMAR, R., HIRST, A. D., *et al* (1991) Increased sensitivity of dopamine receptors and recurrence of affective psychosis after childbirth. *British Medical Journal*, **303**, 613–616.

Further reading

BROCKINGTON, I. (1997) *Motherhood and Mental Health*. Oxford: Oxford University Press.

COX, J. & HOLDEN, J. (eds) (1994) *Aspects of Perinatal Psychiatry – Use and Misuses of the EPDS*. London: Gaskell.

12 Liaison psychiatric services for gynaecological patients

FIONA BLAKE

Gynaecologists and general practitioners are aware that many women attending their clinics with gynaecological complaints are anxious and distressed. There are many cogent reasons why gynaecological complaints are linked with a woman's psychological well-being. They are associated with her femininity, sexuality, attractiveness, physical integrity, bodily functions, moods, life transitions, roles in life and her intimate relationships.

Patterns of presentation

There are several patterns of presentation that may appear in the clinic:

(a) distress secondary to a gynaecological disorder, such as cervical cancer;

(b) psychological disorder presenting under the guise of gynae-cological complaint, for example depressive illness presenting as a premenstrual syndrome (PMS);

(c) psychological disorder *and* gynaecological disorder, which may or may not have a common aetiology, such as endometriosis and anxiety disorder;

(d) intolerance of certain gynaecological events in the setting of particular social and relationship stressors, for example complaint of menorrhagia after stopping the oral contraceptive pill following marital breakdown.

In presenting gynaecological complaints, the woman is aware that she will be questioned about intimate details of her life and may require an internal examination. This prospect itself can engender intense anxiety and apprehension. The clinic situation may remind her of other aversive experiences – perhaps the pain and powerlessness of childhood sexual abuse, the shame of teasing about her female parts, critical comments about her size and shape. Sometimes it is a fear originating from an earlier medical experience when the clinician was rough, suggestive or dismissive, especially in the conduct of a vaginal examination or during childbirth.

The presentation may be associated with fears about value judgements that may be made by the clinician because of cultural and moral aspects of the problem, as with termination of pregnancy or sexually transmitted disease.

Surveys show that when women attending a gynaecology clinic are assessed for psychiatric disorder, many of them are shown to have symptoms of a depressive illness or related disorder (Worsley *et al*, 1977). In one study of general gynaecological patients, 46% of women attending had symptoms of affective disorder (Byrne, 1984). Most gynaecological conditions have psychological disorders commonly associated with them and some are inevitably associated with stress and distress. However, if psychiatric disorder *per se* is not considered, then further physical treatments may be pursued that are unnecessary and potentially harmful, and the psychological problem becomes harder to treat.

The rationale for liaison psychiatric input

It is evident that offering a listening ear and giving some explanation of the physiological patterns are important in helping women to cope with gynaecological events. These events may be highly abnormal, such as gynaecological cancer or menorrhagia with anaemia, or within normal limits but hard to bear, such as menopausal symptoms or PMS. Women often feel confused, isolated and anxious when they do not know what is happening to their bodies. It can be enormously helpful to talk through the problems and make some sense of them. Gynaecologists do some of this supportive work but are usually ill-equipped to identify or manage more complex emotional distress and disorder in their patients. Even those who are interested and have good communication skills do not have the time or specialist training to offer the psychological treatments that some patients need. A liaison service will take referrals of women with complex psychological difficulties, but will also educate the referrers so that they improve their own skills in such matters. In most services, overall clinical effectiveness could be enhanced by adequate liaison psychiatry support.

Gynaecological conditions particularly associated with psychiatric morbidity

Menopause

As the menopause approaches, about 20% of women will have symptoms that prompt them to seek medical help. Research shows that the core symptoms associated with the menopause are sweats, flushes and vaginal dryness. These symptoms respond most consistently to hormone replacement therapy (Dennerstein *et al*, 1979; Greene, 1984). Many other symptoms have been linked to hormonal decline but the association is less clear.

In the past it was believed that the menopause was associated with an increase of major depressive illness ('involutional melancholia'). In fact there is no increase of major psychiatric illness, nor of admissions to hospital with affective illness at the menopause (Winokur, 1973). However, women seeking medical help for their symptoms do have a higher rate of psychiatric illness (Ballinger, 1975). In one specialised clinic, women receiving oestrogen implants had a rate of psychiatric disorder of 87% (Montgomery *et al*, 1987). Low mood, insomnia and tiredness secondary to vasomotor symptoms are likely to improve with hormone replacement therapy. Depressive illness is not (Pearce *et al*, 1995).

As well as major depression, many women experience symptoms because of increasing stresses in their lives at the time of the menopause. They may feel responsible for elderly parents, worry about children leaving home, feel uncertain about job security, or fear growing old. The physical changes may cause worry about health and looks and reduce resilience to stress. These issues may interfere with acceptance and response to hormone replacement therapy.

Services for menopausal women will be more effective if emotional problems that are not purely hormonal can be identified and treated appropriately. A liaison service encourages the gynaecologist to address these issues, with backup available if a complex problem is revealed.

Premenstrual syndrome

Many women have fluctuating symptoms and attribute their difficulties to PMS. However, only a small proportion of women who present complaining of PMS actually have 'pure PMS', that is, symptoms that are only premenstrual and that can be confirmed by a prospective daily symptom diary and occur in the absence of other disorders. 'Pure PMS' implies an association with the hormonal changes of the menstrual cycle. Women who have other patterns of symptoms or random fluctuation of symptoms may not realise that their problems are not entirely associated with their menstrual cycle. They may prefer to think of the symptoms as hormonal and therefore medical, rather than psychological or social. This is determined by cultural attitudes and expectations. Depression, anxiety, eating disorders, relationship problems and adjustment difficulties are among the disorders that may be detected among these sufferers. One study found that 59% of a sample of women complaining of PMS had anxiety or depressive disorder (Fava *et al*, 1992).

Some women may not have a completely random pattern of symptoms, but find that premenstrual changes, while not large in themselves, exacerbate underlying difficulties and make them overwhelming premenstrually (Sampson, 1989). Sometimes the psychological issues are more subtle, with premenstrual changes interacting with personality style to produce distress and difficulties in coping.

It is important to consider whether tackling general, persistent stressors may have more benefit than reducing the monthly fluctuation. Whatever treatment is offered for PMS, it should be accompanied by education about the normal changes of the menstrual cycle. In trials, the antidepressant fluoxetine has been shown to relieve PMS (Steiner *et al*, 1995). It has the advantage that it also treats comorbid depressive illness and is well tolerated. A trial of cognitive therapy for PMS has shown significant relief of symptoms compared with a waiting group (Blake *et al*, 1995).

It is not surprising that so much psychiatric morbidity appears in women with PMS. Mostly, the primary complaints are psychological (low mood, anxiety and irritability). It is an acceptable complaint for a multitude of stresses, distress and dissatisfaction, which have usually persisted for some time before presentation. Often the woman seeks help because things have got worse. This is commonly a depressive illness or adjustment reaction to further stress, which has reduced coping. The support of a liaison service can help the gynaecologist deal with women whose PMS complaint is not cyclical; the service can assess and treat severe psychological disorders that have been uncovered.

Chronic pelvic pain

Many women who present with pelvic pain find relief with a normal course of investigation and treatment. There will be some who have chronic pathology, such as endometriosis or pelvic inflammatory disease, which is more of a challenge to control. These women may find their symptoms distressing and sometimes become depressed as a result. Antidepressants or counselling may be more effective than further surgery or analgesia (see Chapter 8) and a liaison service can assist the gynaecologist in the assessment of such patients. Another group of women continue to have symptoms in the face of minimal or absent pathology. These women may have somatisation disorder and have often presented to gastroenterologists with bowel problems as well. Iatrogenic symptoms may complicate this further.

Women with chronic pelvic pain are more likely to have experienced childhood sexual or physical abuse than women with other gynaecological problems and are frequently seen as difficult to treat. Some of these women are depressed and improve considerably when treated with antidepressants. Others have always experienced abdominal pain in response to stress. This becomes pathologised when such a patient is suspected of having an ectopic pregnancy or pelvic inflammatory disease, and embarks on a road of investigation and treatment, sometimes ending in major surgery. A few women find the process a means of obtaining nurture and care that were absent in their early life.

Liaison services can work with gynaecologists to identify women with psychological needs. Those with somatisation or hypochondriasis require specialist help. They are difficult and confusing patients and take up a good deal of time and resources. Treatment consists of engaging the woman in a psychological model and also working with her carers to limit investigations and treatments that may add to, rather than relieve, the problems (Glover & Pearce, 1995).

Sexual problems

Sexual problems are often presented to gynaecologists or are revealed in the course of the assessment and treatment of other gynaecological problems. Dyspareunia, especially associated with abdominal pain, may present as part of a condition such as endometriosis. At the menopause, painful intercourse is associated with dryness and thinning of the vagina and is relieved by hormone replacement therapy. Low libido may also be presented with the hope that hormonal adjustment will help.

Sexual problems may respond to the resolution of physical disorder, but in many cases it is the relationship of the couple that is crucial to the genesis and maintenance of the difficulties. Psychiatric disorder in either partner can diminish sexual interest.

Some women find it difficult to relax sexually. The resulting vaginismus makes penetration painful or impossible. The woman feels embarrassed and a failure, and is consequently more tense next time.

Women who have experienced unwanted or inappropriate sexual activity, particularly in childhood, are especially likely to have sexual problems and blame themselves for difficulties in a sexual relationship in adulthood. Couple counselling and cognitive–behavioural therapy are among the psychological treatments that can help with these psychosexual problems (Hawton, 1985). Gynaecologists are not equipped to deal with these needs and are grateful for help in deciding what management is appropriate.

Infertility

The pleasure and pride of parenthood is regarded as the right of any couple. The inability to conceive is now regarded as a treatable disorder and the couple embark on a roller-coaster ride of hope and disappointment. This process, unless fairly brief, tests the couple's personal resources and can result in psychological difficulties and strain on a relationship that any other demand would have left intact. Fertility organisations appreciate the stress of treatment and have a network of counsellors trained for this work. The providers of *in vitro* fertilisation services are required to provide a counsellor for couples undergoing treatment. Counselling services for other fertility services are patchy and do not always effectively help the gynaecologist to minimise the trauma of interventions. It is desirable that the couple facing the challenge of fertility treatment are supported by a team that works together to meet their physical and psychological needs.

Termination of unwanted pregnancy

There is always a moral dilemma involved in the decision to have a termination. The psychological demands of this decision are usually left to the family and general practitioner to support. Most women will cope with a pragmatic approach, which minimises the decision to a rational choice that is the least of the evils. There is no overall increase in psychiatric morbidity after termination compared with those proceeding with an unplanned pregnancy (Gilchrist *et al*, 1995). For some women, however, the procedure is laden with meaning and is an agonised decision. The procedure can be followed by grief or depression if the woman is very unhappy with her decision or it has awakened past experiences of loss. In the future, guilt may gnaw away, and may be heightened if there are fertility problems or other losses. Depressive illness may be precipitated. Counselling may enable a woman to come to terms with her choice (Gardner & Davidson, 1993). A liaison service can help gynaecologists to identify and refer women who would benefit from such psychological help.

Hysterectomy

The womb is often regarded by a woman as the focus of her femininity and fertility. Even when her family is complete, she may be anxious when hysterectomy is contemplated. She may fear losing her capacity to have more children and also be anxious about whether her sexuality will be diminished. It used to be thought that these issues resulted in an experience of loss that precipitated depression in women after hysterectomy. In fact, research showed that these women had a very high level of psychiatric morbidity *before* the hysterectomy (for benign gynaecological disorder) and that this was probably associated with the misery and distress of chronic menorrhagia, anaemia and pain. After the hysterectomy, psychiatric problems were much reduced, but at 18 months psychiatric morbidity was still higher than in the general population, indicating that some women had more than gynaecological problems (Gath *et al*, 1982).

Women with cancer will also have issues to face that require psychological support and their difficulties can be complicated by psychiatric disorder. Satisfactory psychiatric management is enhanced by access to good liaison services.

Models of liaison services to gynaecology

A variety of models have been proposed for liaison psychiatry services (Royal College of Physicians & Royal College of Psychiatrists, 1995). The service can be well structured and sophisticated, with a multi-disciplinary team involved in teaching, research and policy making as well as providing patient care. This type of service is usually part of an academic department. The Medical Research Council's Department for Reproductive Biology is an example of such a team. In London, academic psychologists play a greater role in providing psychological services to gynaecology.

Specialist clinics are set up to offer help in the management of particularly complex disorders. Their value lies in the availability of specific, up-to-date expertise in a relatively narrow field. They often serve a wide area and the concentration of difficult cases allows research into the chosen disorders. These clinics also provide an opportunity for teaching and training in the particular field.

There are few specialist clinics for psychological problems associated with gynaecology. Services often develop piecemeal, according to interest and the history of the hospital. In Oxford, a service was set up four years ago with myself, a psychiatrist who works closely with the menopause/PMS clinic. My special interest is in psychological aspects of PMS and the menopause. I work from within a well developed liaison service at the John Radcliffe Hospital, but when I arrived links with gynaecology were tenuous. A social worker offers counselling to women considering termination and will also see other women in the gynaecology ward. She is funded by the general hospital trust. Another psychiatrist employed by the general hospital runs a psycho-oncology service and a general psychiatrist sees a few patients with psychosexual problems. Recently, a psychologist has joined the liaison service. She has begun to work in the endometriosis/pelvic pain clinic to support the gynaecologists and teach them skills in the initial management of such patients. She also sees a few of the more complex patients for psychological treatment. Gradually, interest has increased. A recent initiative is the employment of a fertility counsellor. Funding has been secured by the gynaecology department and is administered by the mental health trust.

Conclusions

When women present with gynaecological problems, management will be enhanced by an appreciation of their psychological needs. Some women have psychological disorders secondary to gynaecological pathology or dysfunction. Others have psychological problems disguised as gynaecological problems. Some have coexisting difficulties.

Gynaecologists should appreciate that their procedures and investigations can be distressing and damaging in their own right. Improving sensitivity and skill in listening to women's views may avoid unnecessary distress and reduce the likelihood of complaints. Some of the morbidity encountered is beyond the time and skill available to the gynaecologist and requires psychological or psychiatric assessment and treatment. Close links with a psychiatric liaison service can encourage appropriate referral while also improving understanding of psychological issues among gynaecologists, so that they can risk engaging with the emotional issues presented by the patient and avoid unnecessary investigation and treatment with more confidence.

References

BALLINGER, C. B. (1975) Psychiatric morbidity in the menopause: screening of a general population sample. *British Medical Journal, iii*, 344–346.

BLAKE, F., GATH, D. & SALKOWSKIS, P. (1995) Psychological aspects of premenstrual syndrome. In *Treatment of Functional Somatic Symptoms* (eds R. Mayou, C. Bass & M. Sharpe), pp. 271–284. Oxford: Oxford University Press.

BYRNE, P. (1984) Psychiatric morbidity in a gynaecological clinic: an epidemiological study. *British Journal of Psychiatry*, **144**, 28–34.

DENNERSTEIN, L., BURROWS, G. D., HYMAN, G. J., *et al* (1979) Hormone therapy and affect. *Maturitas*, **1**, 247–259.

FAVA, M., PEDRAZZI, F., GUARALDI, G. P., *et al* (1992) Comorbid anxiety and depression among patients with late luteal dysphonic disorder. *Journal of Anxiety Disorders*, **6**, 325–335.

GARDNER, K. & DAVIDSON, L. (1993) Unwanted pregnancy and abortion. In *Women's Problems in General Practice* (ed. A. McPherson), pp. 120–151. Oxford: Oxford University Press.

GATH, D., COOPER, P. & DAY, A. (1982) Hysterectomy and psychiatric disorder: I. Levels of psychiatric morbidity before and after hysterectomy. *British Journal of Psychiatry*, **140**, 335–350.

GILCHRIST, A. C., HANNAFORD, P., FRANK, P., *et al* (1995) Termination of pregnancy and psychiatric morbidity. *British Journal of Psychiatry*, **167**, 243–248.

GLOVER, L. & PEARCE, S. (1995) Chronic pelvic pain. In *Treatment of Functional Somatic Symptoms* (eds R. Mayou, C. Bass & M. Sharpe), pp. 313–327. Oxford: Oxford University Press.

GREENE, J. G. (1984) *The Social and Psychological Origins of the Climacteric Syndrome*. Aldershot: Gower.

HAWTON, K. (1985) *Sex Therapy: A Practical Guide*. Oxford: Oxford University Press.

MONTGOMERY, J. C., APPLEBY, L., BRINCAT, M., *et al* (1987) Effect of oestrogen and testosterone implants on psychological disorders in the climacteric. *Lancet*, **i**, 297–299.

PEARCE, J., HAWTON, K. & BLAKE, F. (1995) Psychological and sexual symptoms associated with the menopause and the effects of hormone replacement therapy. *British Journal of Psychiatry*, **67**, 163–173.

ROYAL COLLEGE OF PHYSICIANS & ROYAL COLLEGE OF PSYCHIATRISTS (1995) *The Psychological Care of Medical Patients: Recognition of Need and Service Provision*. (College Report CR 35). London: Royal College of Physicians & Royal College of Psychiatrists.

SAMPSON, G. A. (1989) Premenstrual syndrome. *Baillière's Clinical Obstetrics and Gynaecology*, **3**, 687–704.

STEINER, M., STEINBERG, S., STEWART, D., *et al* (1995) Fluoxetine in the treatment of premenstrual dysphoria. *New England Journal of Medicine*, **332**, 1529–1534.

WINOKUR, G. (1973) Depression in the menopause. *American Journal of Psychiatry*, **130**, 92–93.

WORSLEY, A., WALTERS, W. A. W. & WOOD, E. C. (1977) Screening for psychological disturbance amongst gynaecology patients. *Australian and New Zealand Journal of Obstetrics and Gynaecology*, **17**, 214.

13 Liaison psychiatry in the surgical unit

TREVOR FRIEDMAN

This chapter examines the organisation of a psychiatric service for surgical patients. The importance of psychological factors in the management of surgical patients has been highlighted by a report on the psychological care of surgical patients by a joint working party of the Royal College of Surgeons of England and Royal College of Psychiatrists (1997). The changes in recent years in surgical practice, such as endoscopic surgery, the move towards more day-case operations and the shortened length of hospital stays, have to be considered in the organisation of a liaison psychiatry service, although it is unclear whether these changes in surgical practice have had an effect upon psychological morbidity. It is becoming increasingly important to consider the presence of psychological or social factors that may delay the discharge of patients in order to ensure the efficient use of resources.

What are the common problems for liaison psychiatry?

While some psychological problems are commonly seen in general hospital patients, some are specific to surgery, and certain conditions relate to particular areas of surgical intervention.

Pre-operative anxiety

A certain level of apprehension is normal before surgery. The development of panic disorder or transient refusal of surgery is estimated to occur in 5% of general surgery patients (Strain, 1985). These problems frequently arise in people with pre-existing anxiety disorders. There are occasional patients whose phobic anxiety of hospitals or operations is sufficient to prevent them from having essential operations. Treatment with education, anxiety management and short-term tranquilliser use is normally sufficient to deal with these. The concern may relate particularly to a fear of the anaesthetic – the patient is fearful of not waking after the operation or of being paralysed but aware during the operation. These patients normally respond to a cognitive–behavioural approach, combined with education from an interested anaesthetist.

Patients with needle phobia may also need a cognitive–behavioural treatment, using similar techniques to those employed for diabetics with the same problem. There is evidence that behavioural and cognitive interventions designed for pre-operative use lead to reduced anxiety, improved cooperation and less postoperative analgesia, and help to shorten the hospital stay (Horne *et al*, 1994).

Psychiatric disorder

There is a need for the psychiatric management of patients with known mental illness who require surgical intervention. These may range from people with personality disorders and anxiety to people with severe mental illness, such as patients with schizophrenia. Medical and nursing staff on the ward may well be anxious about treating these patients, but this can normally be managed through education. Psychiatric nurse liaison may be important in devising a nursing care plan for these patients.

Alcohol dependence – with the risk of withdrawal symptoms after surgery – is a common problem, as it may cause a confusional state, and it is important to assess alcohol intake pre-operatively rather than when the patient is withdrawing postoperatively, as it may then be more difficult to obtain a history of excessive alcohol consumption.

Psychotropic medication

There may be need for the liaison psychiatrist to provide advice about any possible interactions between the anaesthetic and psychotropic medication, particularly monoamine oxidase inhibitors and lithium. There is also the common problem of patients' psychotropic medication being stopped after admission, when the junior doctor fails to continue it.

It is important that some brief screening for anxiety, previous mental illness, alcohol consumption and use of psychotropic medication forms part of a normal pre-operative assessment. The management of the majority of the problems identified should be by the surgical team, with occasional advice from or referral to specialist psychiatric services.

Consent

There will be occasional patients who are acutely psychiatrically unwell and requiring an operation. The commonest situation in which this occurs in our service involves patients with acute psychoses who have tried to kill themselves by violent means and need urgent surgical repair. Patients may be unable to give meaningful consent or be refusing surgical intervention. The issue of consent to surgery is not covered by the Mental Health Act and operations are allowable only if within the scope of the common law (see Chapter 6). A psychiatric examination will help in the assessment of mental capacity, will help to detail the mental state and will allow advice to be offered on management. The Mental Health Act may need to be invoked should the patient subsequently refuse psychiatric care or is insistent on leaving hospital and in need of further assessment or treatment of the mental disorder.

A few patients refuse consent without obvious signs of mental illness, such as patients with chronic illness facing major surgery, for example diabetics who are blind and in renal failure requiring amputations because of arterial disease. An opinion should be sought to exclude depressive illness or other mental illness as a cause for the refusal.

Consultations regarding surgical in-patients

There is obviously an enormous range of problems that may be seen. It is helpful to have a summary of the more common reasons for referral. The following examples are not meant to comprise an exhaustive list. A knowledge of the range of potential problems can be helpful when discussing services with surgical colleagues. Discussion of these conditions and how they are presently being managed is a useful preliminary to further joint working. This can lead to auditing of the surgical service for the presence of such problems and then to the establishment of a service to improve the quality of care for patients with these conditions.

The European Consultation Liaison Psychiatry Workgroup (Huyse *et al*, 1996) carried out a one-year study of all in-patient referrals from a large number of hospitals across Europe. There were 14 707 referrals assessed in this study, 1684 (11.4%) from surgical services. In the UK centres there were 127 (10.1%) surgical referrals from a total of 1259 patients referred from general hospital wards. Surgical

referrals can be seen to contribute only a small proportion of the
workload to liaison psychiatry services.

The most common sources of surgical referrals to liaison psychiatry
in the UK involved gastrointestinal surgery (29%), self-inflicted injury
(15%), trauma (11%) and cancer surgery (11%). The most common
reasons were for referral were for an assessment of the patient's
psychiatric state (41%) and to assess or manage patients with
unexplained physical symptoms (17%), after a suicide attempt (16%)
or with substance misuse (10%). Smaller numbers of patients were
referred owing to concerns about their coping abilities or a psychiatric
history, assessment of their capacity to give consent or because they
complied poorly with treatment. A similar pattern of referrals was
seen across Europe.

The most common psychiatric diagnoses among the UK surgical
patients were depressive illness (21%), alcohol misuse (12%) and
delirium (11%); 9% were felt not to have a psychiatric disorder.
Among non-surgical referrals the most common diagnoses were
depressive illness (23%), alcohol misuse (8%), delirium (5%) and
anxiety disorders (5%); 16% had no psychiatric disorder.

General surgery

Liaison with breast units is important because of the wide range of
problems associated with breast cancer. These include body image
disturbance following mastectomy, grief and loss relating to mastectomy and diagnosis of cancer, sexual adjustment, cancer issues, and
development of depressive illness. Many breast services have employed 'breast counsellors', but they are often trained in counselling
about breast prostheses and surgical recovery rather than in dealing
with psychological problems. Depressive illness is common after
breast cancer, occurring in a quarter of women in the year following
mastectomy, and there should be services to detect and treat this
(Maguire *et al*, 1978).

Stomach and duodenal surgery are common sources of psychiatric
pathology, with problems commonly related to alcohol misuse and
anxiety disorders. Oesophageal surgery has similar associations with
alcohol misuse and there may be small numbers of patients with
globus with underlying anxiety or eating disorders. Surgical referrals
from patients with other disturbances of the small or large bowel
may also be related to alcohol misuse or eating disorders.

Between 600 and 1000 patients with functional bowel disease or
irritable bowel disease are seen by doctors each week in the UK (Royal
College of Physicians, 1984), and some of these will progress to surgery.

The management of these patients with pain of unknown origin needs close communication between the surgeons and psychiatrists. There are also small but important numbers of referrals from more specialised areas. There are occasional patients with secondary disorders such as psychosis, and mood and anxiety disorders related to thyroid and parathyroid surgery. There are similar infrequent referrals related to disorders due to phaeochromocytoma, Cushing's disease or hyperadrenalism (e.g. anxiety, panic and depression in patients undergoing adrenal gland surgery).

Patients may also be seen after surgery for an acute abdomen with the initial stages of post-traumatic stress disorder related to the experience of the initial injury.

Cardiothoracic surgery

Cardiac surgery is commonly associated with more anxiety than other surgery because of the extra significance of the heart as a vital organ. On occasion the question of compliance with medication or risk of future illness in patients with a history of severe mental illness may be important in deciding upon the patient's suitability for operation. This is particularly important for procedures such as heart transplantation. There is increased importance with these patients of the assessment of agitation or confusion pre-operatively, which may be caused by medication, inadequate pain control or anxiety relating to the operation. These conditions are important to treat pre-operatively as they may be life-threatening postoperatively in individuals with limited cardiac reserve.

Acute confusional states are common and postoperative delirium in patients undergoing major cardiac procedures may persist beyond the third day. Delirium is also reported in up to 70% of proposed cardiotomy patients (Marvinac *et al*, 1991).

There are also high rates of neuropsychological changes after cardiac surgery. It is not clear what the cause of this is, as magnetic resonance studies have not shown new cerebral lesions. The changes may be due to micro-emboli in the early postoperative stages.

Depression is common following coronary artery bypass grafts and there has been interest in cardiac rehabilitation in helping people return to work and other activities after surgery (Mayou & Bryant, 1993). A major problem in organising such courses is that the patients who most need this treatment and are depressed are often those who fail to attend. A system of routine screening after surgery to identify those patients with psychological morbidity is a more efficient way of managing this problem.

Orthopaedic surgery

Routine orthopaedic surgery is frequently performed on elderly patients, who are at particular risk of developing psychiatric problems. An important study by Strain *et al* (1991) involved systematic screening of elderly patients with hip fractures and case referral to the liaison psychiatry service. They examined over 450 patients and showed that with systematic screening for psychiatric disorder they not only reduced the mean length of stay but that this screening led to the earlier detection of psychiatric illness, better psychiatric treatment and substantial cost savings.

Patients involved in acute trauma, who are frequently managed on orthopaedic wards, are at risk of developing post-traumatic stress disorder. Prolonged hospital stays due to severe trauma mean that this condition should often be detected and treated on the surgical ward. This is another opportunity for joint working between surgical and psychiatric medical and nursing staff. The general nurses can include the recognition of post-traumatic stress disorder as part of their nursing plan and can develop some expertise in recognising the symptoms.

Burns units

The history of psychiatric involvement in the management of burns patients dates from the Second World War and the use of group psychotherapy in managing servicemen with disfiguring burns.

There is often a need for early assessment – in the first two or three days after the burn occurs. The patient may be lucid and may be able to give a history of the events leading up to the burn, which may involve mental illness or alcoholism. Patients may be in great pain and be frightened about the possibility of dying or of a severe, mutilating injury. This is not a reasonable time to carry out psychological debriefing for post-traumatic stress disorder but risk factors and information can be gathered for later management.

Patients may stay in burns units for long periods, receiving skin grafts and other surgical interventions. They may remain in pain and have difficulty adjusting to their burns and the effects they can have on their lives. As well as adjustment reactions they may be developing post-traumatic stress disorder and intervention can begin while the patient is in hospital. A smaller number of patients have longer-term problems adjusting while out of hospital and may need further help dealing with their disfigurement and anxiety related to this. Patients with post-traumatic stress disorder need detailed programmes, often involving desensitisation to the triggers causing flashbacks and episodes of anxiety.

Cosmetic surgery

There has been debate about the availability of plastic surgery as part of the National Health Service and this has led to certain health authorities not agreeing to fund any cosmetic surgery. The decision to operate is normally based upon a consideration of the degree of physical deformity and psychological disturbance. Psychological services may be involved in the screening of patients to determine whether they will psychologically benefit from operations.

A project in Leicester has been screening patients requesting cosmetic surgery for three years and has seen over 600 patients. The screening, mostly performed by specialist psychiatric nurses, has mainly been of people requesting breast enlargement, breast reduction, abdominoplasty and rhinoplasty. It often leads to the identification of secondary problems relating to social avoidance, and specific cognitive–behavioural treatment plans can be organised before operation to ensure patients gain maximum benefit from surgery. There are small numbers of patients with serious mental illness or dysmorphophobia who can be identified by the screening process and prevented from having unnecessary operations. The results from this study and explanatory notes are shown in Table 13.1.

TABLE 13.1
Surgical priority for patients screened for plastic surgery

	High priority	Medium priority	Low priority	Others	Total
Rhinoplasty	6	23	6	13	48
Breast enlargement	11	60	4	9	84
Breast reduction	6	99	4	8	117
Abdominoplasty	9	54	3	10	76
Tattoo removal	2	5	0	6	13
Maxillofacial	1	6	0	1	8
Ears	4	19	4	8	35
Liposuction	3	5	1	0	9
Miscellaneous	5	11	3	6	25
Total	47	282	25	61	415

High-priority and medium-priority patients are those felt to be suffering major psychological distress who would benefit from surgery. Those with low priority would benefit from surgery but are not sufficiently distressed to warrant treatment on the National Health Service. 'Others' did not attend for screening or were suffering from other psychiatric illnesses in which surgery would be contraindicated.

The study showed approximately 20% of patients screened were not felt to be appropriate for surgery. This was either because they were not felt to be in sufficient distress (6%), had other psychiatric problems, or did not attend for assessment (15%). Operations most likely to be approved were breast enlargement (85%), breast reduction (90%) and abdominoplasty (83%). Those least likely to be approved were rhinoplasty (60%), tattoo removals (54%), ear operations (66%) and miscellaneous requests (64%). In understanding these figures it must be remembered that these patients have gone through a process of selection already via their general practitioner before referral and so would be expected to show high levels of morbidity.

Outcome data on the first 100 patients in terms of psychological, social and sexual functioning indicate dramatic improvements following surgery. A large number of patients who have had surgery and those found to be suffering from psychiatric illnesses have benefited from psychiatric treatment. This has been to help them with problems of anxiety, evident as social withdrawal, depression, disturbances of body image (dysmorphophobia) and sexual difficulties. The screening has proved extremely valuable in validating the practice of plastic surgeons as well as providing better psychological care for this group of patients. It also provides a model of how a study can lead to greater liaison, as the purchasers become aware of the greater overall quality of care that may be offered with psychiatric liaison.

Head and neck surgery

The major specific difficulties encountered here are associated with the severely disfiguring surgery carried out on people's faces. Patients are helped by a programme of education before surgery, which includes the family. Self-help groups can be beneficial in supporting people through this difficult time.

Elderly surgical patients

Acute confusional states are the most common psychiatric disorder encountered in elderly patients in the general hospital. They are found in 15% of elderly surgical patients, and this incidence rises to 30% of postcardiotomy patients and to 50% of postoperative hip fracture patients. They are a marker of illness severity, a poor prognostic sign and a sign that further investigations are required

(Roca, 1994). Experience indicates that delirium is frequently unrecognised and under-treated.

Dementia increases in prevalence with age, and rates are higher in institutional settings such as nursing homes and hospitals. Admission to hospital may reveal an underlying dementia, which may be exacerbated by delirium. Recognition of dementia at the time of admission leads to better management and the planning of care after discharge. The Mini Mental State Examination is a simple measure that can be used routinely to screen elderly patients for cognitive impairment (Folstein *et al*, 1975).

Depression is common in general hospitals and is often under-diagnosed and under-treated (Katon, 1987), largely because of a misconception that the distress is understandable and related to the patient's condition (Rifkin, 1992); this is probably even more true of surgical patients. The recognition of depressive illness in elderly patients can be improved by the use of screening measures such as the Geriatric Depression Scale (Yesavage *et al*, 1983).

Out-patient consultations

Out-patient referrals from surgeons reflect the pattern of in-patient referrals, although with less organic brain syndromes and more patients with unexplained pain and other symptoms. Services need to decide whether they accept referrals of patients with surgical problems from general practitioners or restrict themselves only to requests from general hospital specialists.

Organisation of the service

The evidence from studies, as mentioned earlier, is that the majority of referrals for liaison psychiatry are from physicians rather than surgeons. This may be because of differences between surgeons and physicians, in surgical patients or in the surgical process. Surgeons may be less well trained in this respect, or temperamentally less interested in identifying mental illness. Surgeons may not feel that dealing with these problems comes within their remit, in rather the same way as they would not manage a myocardial infarction or diabetes. There is evidence from work in the management of cancer patients that lack of confidence in managing psychological problems leads to an avoidance of picking up cues from patients that they are distressed. There may be lower rates of psychiatric morbidity in surgical patients but there is no evidence to support this. The patients may be less likely to discuss psychological problems with surgeons than with other doctors. There is an aura around the whole process of surgery that influences patients' expectations and results in large placebo effects (Johnson, 1994). The routine management or 'processing' of non-emergency elective surgery may lead to less opportunity for discussion with the doctor about psychological problems. It seems likely that day patients may not be so thoroughly assessed as in-patients regarding their psychosocial problems.

It is apparent from the difficulties noted above that there is often a need for education and training of surgeons in the recognition and management of psychological problems. This can be very difficult to achieve. The use of screening questionnaires can be helpful but there is often a reluctance to include extra paperwork and there is then the larger problem of managing the patients who score above the threshold on such measures.

An important role of the liaison psychiatrist is to raise the awareness of mental illness within general hospitals, to obtain better management for patients. It is unlikely that many surgeons will attend lectures on the detection and management of mental illness in their patients and so other opportunities have to be explored. Individual consultants may refer only one or two patients a year, presumably because these patients were particularly challenging or exceptional in some way. This may be that surgeon's only contact with psychiatry and it is therefore important that they are kept informed by copy letters on the progress of the patient. Success with an individual patient can be highly effective in changing a surgeon's view of psychiatry and there can be frustration if the surgeon is not informed of the patient's outcome.

There are opportunities to present cases at grand rounds or surgical meetings. Experience suggests that such offers are normally enthusiastically received by surgeons. It is particularly helpful if psychiatric aspects of an illness can be included as part of a study day covering other aspects of the illness (pathology, pharmacology, etc.) as this helps to lead to an integrated approach by surgeons in managing a particular condition.

There are the established liaison roles in joint clinics or ward rounds. These are undoubtedly an effective way of raising awareness of liaison psychiatry but they are time-consuming and one has to be certain that this is an efficient use of psychiatric time. It may be more useful to spend a limited amount of time with a surgical team, auditing the prevalence of psychiatric morbidity, the impact of psychiatric services and education, followed by a review of future plans. This is also a valuable experience for trainee liaison psychiatrists.

The conditions dealt with by liaison psychiatry demand the ability to respond with a range of treatments, including pharmacological, psychodynamic and cognitive–behavioural. The psychiatric team should reflect these skills. The use of nurse specialists with some of these skills and the ability to gain experience in particular physical conditions can be invaluable.

Links with specific services

It may be possible to move towards links with services which have specific needs. One of the difficulties is that the service depends upon the surgeons being interested in this area of their work; education and joint working may help to raise the awareness of this area. Areas that may particularly benefit from links are burns and plastic surgery units, orthopaedic/trauma units, cardiothoracic units and transplant units.

Problems of workload and contracting

There is often a problem in the UK with the increased workload produced by these links and it is necessary to initiate discussion and agreement concerning how this will be resourced. In Leicester we have a model in which skilled clinical nurse specialists have an involvement in one particular area and as the workload increases they can be funded on a sessional basis by the surgical directorate. This is also beneficial in increasing liaison between psychiatric and general nurses, who are often more involved in the day-to-day management of patients. There can be problems with open-ended 'block' contracts where there is an agreement to see all the patients referred. There is generally a great deal of unrecognised psychiatric morbidity and this can lead to a rapid increase in workload without increased resources. This increase should form part of the contract with the purchasers of psychiatric services.

References

FOLSTEIN, M. F., FOLSTEIN, S. F. & McHUGH, P. R. (1975) The Mini Mental State: a practical method for grading the cognitive state of patients for the clinician. *Journal of Psychiatric Research*, **12**, 189–195.

HORNE, D. L., VATMANADIS, P. & CARERI, A. (1994) Preparing patients for invasive medical and surgical procedures. 1: Adding behavioural and cognitive interventions. *Behavioural Medicine*, **20**, 5–13.

HUYSE, F. J., HERZOG, T., MALT, U. F., *et al* (1996) The European Consultation Liaison Workgroup Collaborative Study. I. General outline. *General Hospital Psychiatry*, **18**, 44–55.

162   *Friedman*

JOHNSON, A. L. (1994) Surgery as a placebo. *Lancet*, **344**, 1140–1142.

KATON, W. (1987) The epidemiology of depression in medical care. *International Journal of Psychiatry*, **17**, 93–112.

MAGUIRE, G. P., LEE, E. O., BEVINGTON, D. J., *et al* (1978) Psychiatric problems in the first year after mastectomy. *British Medical Journal*, **276**, 963–965.

MARVINAC, C. M. (1991) Neurological dysfunctions following cardiac surgery. *Critical Care Nursing in North America*, **3**, 691–698.

MAYOU, R. & BRYANT, B. (1993) Quality of life in cardiovascular disease. *British Heart Journal*, **69**, 460–466.

RIFKIN, A. (1992) Depression in physically ill patients. *Postgraduate Medicine*, **92**, 147–154.

ROCA, R. (1994) Psychosocial aspects of surgical care in the elderly patient. *Surgical Clinics of North America*, **74**, 223–243.

ROYAL COLLEGE OF PHYSICIANS (1984) The need for an increased number of consultant physicians with specialist training in gastroenterology. *Gut*, **25**, 99–102.

ROYAL COLLEGE OF SURGEONS OF ENGLAND & ROYAL COLLEGE OF PSYCHIATRISTS (1997) *Report of the Working Party on the Psychological Care of Surgical Patients*. Council Report CR55. London: Royal College of Surgeons of England/Royal College of Psychiatrists.

STRAIN, J. J. (1985) The surgical patient. In *Psychiatry* (eds R. Michels & J. O. Cazenar), vol. 2, pp. 1–11. Philadelphia: J. B. Manipincott.

——, LYANS, J. S., HAMMER, J. S., *et al* (1991) Cost offset from a psychiatric consultation liaison intervention with elderly hip fracture patients. *American Journal of Psychiatry*, **148**, 1044–1049.

YESAVAGE, J. A., BRINK, T. L. & ROSE, T.L. (1983) Development and validation of a geriatric depression screening scale: a preliminary report. *Journal of Psychiatric Research*, **17**, 37–49.

,

14 Liaison psychiatry in palliative care

JENNIFER BARRACLOUGH

The palliative care setting

Palliative care is defined as:

"the active total care of patients and their families by a multi professional team at a time when the patient's disease is no longer responsive to curative treatment and life expectancy is relatively short. It is patient-focused and not disease-focused. It responds to physical, psychological, social and spiritual needs, and extends if necessary to support in bereavement. The goal of palliative care is to provide support and care for patients in the last phases of the disease so that they can live as fully and comfortably as possible." (Twycross, 1999, p. 2)

Modern palliative care (alternatively termed hospice or terminal care) in the UK dates from 1967, when St Christopher's Hospice, London, opened under the leadership of Dr Cicely Saunders. Palliative medicine became recognised as a medical speciality in 1987. A recent handbook lists 217 in-patient units in the UK and Republic of Ireland (Hospice Information Service, 1996): although most units have close links with the National Health Service (NHS), including joint funding arrangements, about 75% of them are primarily managed and funded by the voluntary and charitable sector.

Staff include specialised doctors, nurses, social workers, occupational therapists, physiotherapists, chaplains, bereavement counsellors, creative and complementary therapists, and volunteers. Training programmes for various professions have been developed and many units have study centres. Research has been slower to evolve, but this is now changing with the establishment of several academic departments and the Palliative Care Research Forum of Great Britain and Ireland.

In the early days of the speciality, medical investigations and treatment were little used, and the emphasis was on caring for those at the very end of life in small in-patient units. Most beds were reserved for patients with cancer, with a few for motor neuron disease. The scope of palliative care has been widened by recent trends in service provision to include:

(a) day centres, community care programmes and general hospital support teams;
(b) emphasis on symptom control and rehabilitation – many patients are now referred well before they reach the terminal stage and about 50% of in-patient episodes end in discharge rather than death;
(c) progressive and incurable medical conditions other than cancer, for example chronic chest disease, heart disease, neurological illnesses and AIDS;
(d) a distinction between 'specialist palliative care' and the more general 'palliative care approach' – not all dying people and their families need specialist palliative care, but the general principles are relevant to the incurable and terminally ill in any health care setting, and this is true for psychiatric as well as physical illness, most obviously in relation to dementia but possibly also to other intractable severe mental disorders;
(e) outreach to ethnic and religious minorities, who have been underrepresented in the past.

The importance of psychosocial aspects of palliative care is widely acknowledged. Accounts of the normal and abnormal psychology of dying and bereavement have come from psychiatrists and others (e.g. Kubler-Ross, 1970; Hinton, 1972; Parkes, 1972; Stedeford & Bloch, 1979; Cassidy, 1986; Lichter, 1991; Ramsay, 1992; Stedeford, 1994).

Psychological reactions to terminal illness

Psychiatric disorders in palliative care patients must be considered in the context of the psychological response to incurable progressive disease. Such a diagnosis may bring a host of losses and fears. Sadness, worry and anger are common reactions, although some patients show surprisingly little emotion and appear to be denying the seriousness of their plight. In most cases, these initial reactions will be replaced within weeks by realistic acceptance of the situation and adaptation to it. This process may be repeated as the disease advances.

The nature and degree of distress for each individual are partly dependent on personality and experience, but also strongly influenced by medical management. Adjustment tends to be difficult for those whose diagnosis has been unduly delayed, who perceive their 'bad news interview' as insensitively handled, or who feel 'written off' by their doctors, with a consequent loss of hope. In contrast, great comfort may come from the assurance that professional interest and support, and active control of symptoms, will continue to be available until the end of life.

Many of those who fulfil diagnostic criteria for depressive illness at this time are experiencing a transient adjustment process, which will resolve without antidepressants, and few need to be seen by a psychiatrist.

Nature and prevalence of psychiatric syndromes

Little systematic research has been published on prevalence rates for psychiatric symptoms in palliative care patients. There are a number of reasons for this:

(a) conventional psychiatric diagnostic criteria are confounded by the somatic symptoms of medical illness and by psychological reactions to dying, and may not be valid or relevant in this population (this issue has been best studied with respect to depression, and is further considered below);
(b) many patients are too unwell to cooperate with any but the briefest of assessments;
(c) the culture of palliative care has encouraged individual description of problems rather than use of standardised interviews or questionnaires, although this is changing with the introduction of quality-of-life (QOL) instruments, which combine measures of psychological, somatic, social and sometimes spiritual well-being.

Depression and anxiety are clearly important, and the Hospital Anxiety and Depression (HAD) Scale (Zigmond & Snaith, 1983) is probably the most widely used instrument for screening palliative care populations. In a large community sample of patients with incurable cancer in London, 30% of patients scored high on the HAD for depression, and 23% scored high for anxiety (Addington-Hall *et al.*, 1992). For in-patients, my personal experience of using the HAD in both Oxford and Southampton indicates that about 25% score high, and 25% score borderline, for depression and anxiety, but that only about 60% of newly admitted patients are well enough to fill in the form. Interview studies also suggest a prevalence of about 25% for clinically significant depression, depending on the criteria chosen (Chochinov *et al.*, 1994). Most cases are mild or moderate; severe depression with psychotic features is rare.

No clear association of mood disorder with age, sex, or medical diagnosis has been found. Probable risk factors include a psychiatric history, poorly controlled pain and other physical symptoms, low physical performance status, presence of organic mental disorders, actual or perceived lack of social support, low self-esteem, adverse life events and social difficulties. However, the multiplicity of factors operating in each individual case rules out accurate predictions of who will be affected. Although some patients with pre-existing psychiatric illness present very difficult management problems when they are terminally ill, others show improvements in mental state at this time.

Organic mental disorders are common, especially in older patients and those very near the end of life. One study (Power *et al*, 1993) found that one-third of new in-patients had cognitive impairment as measured by the Abbreviated Mental Test Score. About 50% of palliative care patients do not have psychiatric symptoms. Some report psychological benefits from their illness experience, for example closer relationships and a clearer sense of their priorities and purpose in life.

Partners and close relatives are also at risk of depression and anxiety, both before and after the death of the patient.

Detection of cases and arrangements for referral

Psychological awareness in palliative care units is greater than in most general hospital settings, but some psychiatric disorders still go undetected because they present with somatic symptoms, or because certain staff are reluctant to ask about emotional issues. Cases which are recognised may be left untreated because they are assumed to represent normal reactions, or because a stigma is felt to attach to mental health referral.

Delays in recognition and referral often mean that patients have become too physically unwell to cooperate with full assessment, let alone to carry a course of treatment through, by the time they meet the psychiatrist. Screening all patients at intervals with a short instrument such as the HAD Scale, as mentioned above, would seem, in theory, the best way to ensure prompt action, but this does not work well in practice unless all staff understand the purpose of the exercise, how to explain it to patients, how to add up the scores and the importance of following up a high score. A more personalised approach, in which potential referrals are discussed with the psychiatrist at unit meetings or by individual staff, may be preferred. Following such discussion, the psychiatrist would either arrange to see the patient in person or offer advice on managing the case.

The suggestion of psychiatric referral often comes from a nurse or other staff member, but it is my own practice to see patients only with the prior agreement of the medical consultant or the general practitioner, and preferably after discussion with other members of the palliative care team. The patient's own agreement is essential and a phrase such as "the doctor on our staff with a special interest in the psychological aspects of illness" usually proves an acceptable introduction.

About 10% of patients coming through the hospice in Oxford (Sobell House) are referred for psychiatric assessment. Some are seen once only for an advisory consultation, others on many occasions until death, whether as in-patients, out-patients or day patients, in the general hospital or at home.

The assessment process

The standard headings of the psychiatric history and mental state examination provide a sound framework for the interview, and use of this comprehensive system of enquiry may well elicit important information which a less structured approach would miss. However, many patients are too sick to answer all the questions, and some sections may be irrelevant, so individual judgement is needed. Establishing nurses' and relatives' views of the problem, reading the medical notes and the drug chart contribute to the assessment.

Being trained in both medical and psychological aspects, the psychiatrist can offer a useful 'fresh look' at a difficult case from a broad perspective. This may result in the diagnosis of a psychiatric disorder, with specific implications for management. Sometimes, however, the making or exclusion of a psychiatric diagnosis is less important than eliciting patients' own concerns and addressing these. Concerns often relate to physical symptoms, body image, family burden, practical matters such as housing and finance, and/or unanswered (and often unanswerable) questions about medical diagnosis, life expectancy, the dying process and the mode of death. Spiritual and existential issues, of a kind which are often not addressed within the practice of mainstream psychiatry, frequently arise.

Reasons for psychiatric referral

The main reasons for psychiatric referral are considered below in approximate order of frequency. Many patients have more than one of these problems.

Depression

Depression accounts for about half of referrals (Billings & Block, 1995). Diagnostic uncertainty is frequent. The key symptoms of clinical depression are psychological ones: sustained low mood over and above understandable sadness, loss of interest, feelings of guilt, worthlessness and hopelessness, suicidal thoughts or behaviour. Somatic symptoms such as insomnia, anorexia and fatigue, although likely to result in part from the medical illness, should not be ignored in the assessment. Even if the diagnosis of depression is in little doubt, advice may be needed on management, because the condition is severe or the first-line drug has failed.

Anxiety and panic attacks

Fears about death and dying probably underlie most cases, although not all patients are able or willing to talk about them. Unacknowledged anxiety may present through exacerbation of somatic symptoms such as pain, nausea and/or breathlessness. Depression may be associated. Overwhelming anxiety towards the end of life forms part of the 'terminal anguish' syndrome of uncontrollable distress and pain.

Organic mental disorders

These are often secondary to the illness itself (e.g. primary brain tumour, cerebral metastases, hypercalcaemia) or to medical treatment (e.g. steroids or other drugs, radiotherapy to the brain) (Breitbart *et al.*, 1995). Other causes include substance misuse, such as alcohol withdrawal, or dementia. Presentations include cognitive impairment, mood change (depression or hypomania), paranoid symptoms, 'personality change', hallucinations and disturbed behaviour. Some of these are easily mistaken for psychogenic reactions. Organic impairments usually exacerbate psychological distress and complicate the process of adjustment to illness, but for some patients they appear to confer a welcome psychological detachment.

Complex adjustment reactions

These occur when patients are unable to come to terms with their medical condition. They may take many forms. Anger may be well justified if the case was genuinely mismanaged, but sometimes anger regarding the illness itself is being displaced against health care staff or family members. Denial, which to some extent is an adaptive psychological defence mechanism, causes problems when present in extreme form. Some patients adopt a passive, helpless stance, which prevents any worthwhile quality of life. Role changes within a family may affect several of its members.

Somatic symptoms

Physical complaints can seldom be attributed to psychological causes alone, but it is common for difficult-to-control pain, nausea, breathlessness or fatigue to have some psychological component. A holistic view is called for, with physical and psychological aspects both being addressed.

Deliberate self-harm

Suicide and self-harm are uncommon clinically, although many palliative care patients have thought about suicide, and patients with cancer have a 1.8-fold increase in suicide rate (Harris & Barraclough, 1994). In the cases I have seen, associated factors include clinical depression, social isolation, reluctance to burden other people, a sense of loss of control in a previously dominant personality and inadequate pain control. Effective interventions for at least some of these problems can almost always be offered.

Partners and close relatives are at increased risk of suicide in the early weeks or months of their bereavement, especially in the presence of depression, alcohol misuse or social difficulties, and if they had a close or complex relationship with the deceased. Vulnerable individuals can usually be identified in advance by the nurses or social workers caring for the patient, and offered support through the bereavement service and the primary care team, with psychiatric referral if indicated.

Miscellaneous referrals

These include troublesome nightmares, sexual problems, post-traumatic stress disorder, severe psychiatric disorder pre-dating the medical illness, and 'difficult' patients whose personalities lead to discord with staff.

Interventions

Diagnosis

Is the patient clinically depressed, or working through an appropriate adjustment reaction, or physically ill? Sometimes the assessment suggests a primarily medical cause for the symptoms, rather than a psychiatric one. Mood changes secondary to corticosteroid medication are common and have usually been recognised by the medical team. Other examples are found: a woman referred because of 'anxiety' was found to be exhibiting motor akathisia, which resolved when the dose of metoclopramide, prescribed to control nausea, was reduced. In other cases the psychiatrist might suggest a medical investigation such as a brain scan. Sometimes the opinion might be that the patient's psychological reaction is within normal limits, given his or her personality and circumstances.

Drug treatment

Psychotropic drugs, including antidepressants, anxiolytics and antipsychotics, are widely prescribed by palliative care physicians, for relief of both psychological and physical symptoms, but psychiatric advice is required for less straightforward cases.

A good response to antidepressant drugs has been observed for about 80% of depressed patients at Sobell House (unpublished audit). This includes some patients with brain tumours. We use amitriptyline as the first-line drug when there is a requirement for sedation or pain relief, and sertraline when there are medical contraindications to tricyclics or a risk of overdose. Some authorities recommend psychostimulants such as methylphenidate as alternatives to conventional antidepressant drugs (Billings & Block, 1995).

Intermittent doses of benzodiazepines are useful for managing anxiety, but are not a substitute for exploring its causes or applying psychological management techniques. Antipsychotics, usually haloperidol or thioridazine, are indicated for agitated or psychotic patients, including those with organic mental disorders. Both benzodiazepines (usually midazolam) and antipsychotics (usually haloperidol) are often prescribed together with opioids by the subcutaneous route in the terminal phase, to help control pain, nausea, agitation and distress.

Long-term medication for a pre-existing psychiatric disorder can often be slowly tapered off in the last few weeks of life, while keeping careful watch for relapse. If psychotic symptoms do persist after the patient has become unable to swallow oral medicines, a depot antipsychotic may be prescribed.

Psychotherapy

Interventions must be brief and flexible. Plans for a set number of regular weekly sessions are frequently impossible to carry through, owing to fluctuations in a patient's physical state, or clashes with medical appointments. The therapy process, and development of transference, is likely to be influenced by concurrent relationships with other staff whose role includes a psychological aspect.

Sometimes only a single assessment interview is possible before the patient dies, but the process of reviewing the story of the illness from a psychological point of view in the context of life history, and ventilation of feelings with a person who is not directly involved in providing medical care, can have a powerful therapeutic effect.

Some dying patients feel a need to explore issues from their past: sexual abuse, trauma in a prisoner-of-war camp, or marital violence by a long-dead spouse. Special techniques such as imagery may help patients work through their fears of dying (Kearney, 1996).

Cognitive–behavioural psychotherapy (Greer & Moorey, 1997) and problem-solving techniques (Wood & Mynors-Wallis, 1997) may be helpful, especially for those who have lost all sense of control over their lives. One man, referred because his depression had not responded to amitriptyline, was noted to be leaving every decision to his loving wife. His mood improved after he had been encouraged to choose his own television viewing and his own menus, and take a daily walk.

Although they may not have a formal psychiatric disorder, some patients with a longer life expectancy claim benefit from ongoing interviews, perhaps about once a month, to review their progress and feelings and talk over treatment decisions. This aspect of the psychiatrist's role could be described as 'companion' to the physically ill (Druss, 1995).

Groups

Groups for this patient population can have a specific focus, such as teaching relaxation or anxiety management, or a less structured 'supportive–expressive' format. A patient support group ran for five years at Sobell House, responsibility being shared between myself and the social worker, with a Macmillan nurse or other colleague as co-facilitator. Despite the repeated experience of loss through death of its members, the group proved a positive experience for both patients and staff. Patients had the opportunity to ventilate their feelings, in a confidential setting, with others who could empathise from their own personal experience and sometimes suggest new ways of coping. It showed the psychiatrist a broader spectrum of psychological reactions than is available from seeing referred patients only. Patients who would benefit from individual referral could often be identified by observing them in the group. Although this was a support group, not a therapy one, it proved important to ensure that all staff involved received training and supervision in the principles of group work and the boundaries to be observed.

Non-psychiatric interventions

Many practical, supportive and complementary interventions are used in palliative care. Such simple things as a new hairstyle, a more comfortable mattress, a trip to a favourite place or a visit from a PAT (Pets as Therapy) dog can bring about big improvements in a patient's emotional well-being and sometimes appear more effective than psychotropic drugs. Referral to an occupational, physio- or creative therapist may permit more specialised techniques to be used, including relaxation training, massage and aromatherapy, and music or art therapy.

Effectiveness of treatment

Devising valid outcome measures for any intervention in palliative care poses a major challenge, because of a number of constraints:

(a) whereas in most other health care settings the death of a patient represents a failure of treatment, in palliative care it is the expected outcome;

(b) there may be individual variation in what outcome is to be considered desirable, depending for example on whether the patient wishes to die at home or in hospital;

(c) many patients do not live long enough for follow-up or, even if they do, may not be well enough to complete any but the simplest of standardised assessments;

(d) the case mix in palliative care settings is heterogeneous;

(e) patients receive several medical and social interventions concurrently, which hampers the evaluation of individual treatments;

(f) there may be ethical barriers to the notion of randomising dying patients in clinical trials.

The most relevant measures, which tend to be qualitative rather than quantitative, have been listed in a report from the National Council for Hospice and Specialist Palliative Care (1995) as those relating to quality of life, quality of dying, family needs and bereavement outcome. This report gives details of several measurement instruments which, with the exception of the HAD Scale, all include a mixture of physical and psychological items.

Because follow-up measures can be obtained with only a minority of patients, few completed trials of psychological treatments have been published. Noble (1996) carried out a study with out-patients who scored high on the HAD Scale; the treatment package of brief counselling, anxiety management training and antidepressant drugs appeared to alleviate physical symptoms but to have little effect on psychological ones. Wood & Mynors-Wallis (1997) found in a pilot study that problem-solving techniques proved acceptable and feasible with palliative care patients.

In clinical practice, most patients referred to a psychiatrist appear to benefit from the intervention, as the following case vignette shows:

A 60-year-old man with locally advanced bowel cancer had been depressed for several months before referral, despite taking 40 mg fluoxetine daily. He complained of severe pain despite various medical interventions. During his four-week in-patient stay on the palliative care ward, his antidepressant was changed to 50 mg amitriptyline at night, gradually raised to 175 mg. This brought about a rapid improvement in his sleep pattern and reduced his anxiety and pain. The psychiatrist visited him two or three times a week on the ward. All his life this patient had found great difficulty in talking about his feelings, but he gradually revealed two main concerns: his fear of death, linked with memories of his father's painful death from cancer some years previously; and his fear of being abandoned by his partner on account of the sexual dysfunction caused by his pelvic disease. Besides ventilation of feelings, the sessions included provision of information about his cancer and its treatment, and encouragement to communicate with his partner. His physical and emotional state improved sufficiently for him to be discharged, with care from a Macmillan nurse and social services. He enjoyed a good quality of life at home for several months before he died.

For occasional patients, psychiatric consultation appears to make matters worse, often by interfering with a defence of denial:

A young woman with complex and longstanding emotional problems had concealed a breast lump for years and presented with an advanced fungating tumour but apparently expecting a cure. The psychiatric assessment interview was long and intensive; although she appeared to find it helpful at the time, she subsequently expressed much anger towards the psychiatrist and cancelled further sessions.

Liaison with colleagues

In contrast to those medical settings in which the liaison psychiatrist may be the only staff member with expertise in psychosocial matters, most palliative care units have some staff who are highly skilled in the psychological management of dying patients and their families. Therefore, in a well functioning unit, there is excellent scope for multi-professional teamwork. However, there is also, especially if communication between team members is inadequate, a risk that excessive overlap will lead to confusion of roles and responsibilities, the overburdening of patients by involvement of multiple staff, and waste of professional time. As well as regular discussion between colleagues, it may be useful to draw up local guidelines to clarify the skills of the different staff available in a particular unit (National Council for Hospice and Specialist Palliative Care, 1997).

After psychiatric assessment, management can frequently be continued by the staff who are already involved, with supervision from the psychiatrist, who may or may not need to review the patient in person again from time to time. At Sobell House, I meet weekly with the ward team, the day centre staff and the Macmillan nursing team to discuss cases already known to me, and new ones which might require either personal referral or advice.

Sometimes, it is the relationship with the caregiving team which needs attention as much as the individual patient's clinical state. Staff may become overinvolved with certain patients, usually younger ones well known to the unit, or with their families. Spending excessive amounts of time with such patients, while neglecting to maintain professional boundaries, can lead to great emotional distress for staff. Conversely, staff may feel frustrated or angered by patients who seem demanding or unappreciative; such responses cannot always be frankly acknowledged within a culture which seeks to maintain the highest ideals of care. Both situations can sometimes be helped by team meetings which include the opportunity for ventilation of feelings. Explanation may help; dealing with a patient's anger is somewhat easier if it is perceived as a symptom of depressive illness or organic brain disease, as opposed to deliberate rudeness. The management plan, agreed by all concerned, should include a consistent approach to the patient and family, and the setting of clear, practical goals. Sometimes no change in management is called for, but it is helpful to make a positive statement that the best possible is already being done and to acknowledge the difficulties the staff are having.

Liaison with the mental health unit is required for patients already under treatment there, and for the very rare cases where severe mental disorder calls for electroconvulsive therapy or for compulsory treatment under the Mental Health Act 1983.

Education and support of colleagues

Educational presentations for staff within the palliative care unit are designed both to help them identify cases needing psychiatric referral and to enhance their own psychological skills. When the right atmosphere is achieved, these events can also fulfil some staff support function. Whether the psychiatrist is the best person to lead a designated 'staff support group' is debatable. It is difficult to find the right formula for such groups, but perhaps ideally they should be led by someone who knows about palliative care but is not a member of the clinical team.

There is a considerable demand for formal training of various groups: medical students, hospital staff (doctors, nurses, radiographers) in palliative care or oncology, general practitioners, psychiatrists and other mental health professionals, and voluntary groups. Topics include psychological reactions to terminal illness, recognition and management of specific psychiatric syndromes (anxiety, depression, organic mental disorders), skills of communication and breaking bad news, the 'difficult patient' and personal support.

Training psychiatrists for work in palliative care

The psychiatrist working in palliative care needs the following:

(a) to know about the medical aspects of palliative care, including drug treatments;
(b) to appreciate the usual range of psychological reactions to terminal illness;
(c) to be prepared to talk openly with patients about dying and death;
(d) to be familiar with the culture of palliative care units;
(e) to be willing to work in a team, and respect the skills of other professionals and volunteers;
(f) to maintain links with mental health services so as to be able to refer cases to other colleagues on occasion, and to avoid professional isolation.

A session about palliative care could usefully be included on courses leading to the membership examination of the Royal College of Psychiatrists, so that all trainees have a basic introduction, and clinical training attachments could be made available for those who are interested. In Oxford, attachments of one session per week have been arranged for several registrars and senior registrars whose main post is in liaison psychiatry, old age psychiatry or psychotherapy. Clinical attachments should not be compulsory, because some psychiatric trainees are temperamentally unsuited to palliative care work, and it is unfair for terminally ill patients to receive their one and only psychiatric assessment from someone without a reasonable level of interest and skill.

Service planning

The importance of psychosocial matters is already widely appreciated by senior colleagues in palliative care. For cancer patients and their families, who still form the majority of those managed in this setting, this has been formally endorsed in the influential 'Calman–Hine report' regarding cancer services in England and Wales (Chief Medical Officer's Expert Advisory Group on Cancers, 1995). However, the widely used term 'psychosocial support' can become a cliché, implying that a broadly caring and sympathetic approach is sufficient on its own. The case for employing a psychiatrist, whose time is expensive and whose involvement may be regarded as carrying a stigma, needs to be justified to planners and purchasers. One common misunderstanding is that psychiatry offers nothing different from counselling or complementary therapy; another is that psychiatrists are concerned only with psychotic patients. Aspects of the psychiatrist's contribution which therefore need to be overtly specified include:

(a) carrying out diagnostic assessments which take account of both medical and psychosocial factors;
(b) identifying specific psychiatric conditions which require specialised treatment;
(c) prescribing psychotropic drug regimens of the more complex kind;
(d) initiating specialised psychological treatments;
(e) supervising and coordinating the psychological work of other staff;
(f) liaising with colleagues in mental health care services;
(g) offering training to a wide range of professionals.

Benefits of the service are not confined to those patients treated in person and should be viewed more broadly, in terms of formal and informal education of colleagues in the general hospital, in primary care, in mental health units and in other settings about this aspect of the palliative care approach. Justification for the service cannot be adequately presented in quantitative terms. As discussed above, both assessment of needs and evaluation of outcomes are complicated for palliative care patients. Although there is good evidence for a substantial prevalence of depression and other psychiatric disorders in this population, with reliable figures to be quoted, evidence for the effectiveness of treatment is, inevitably, harder to come by. Measurements developed for other health care settings often appear inappropriate in this context. They certainly cannot do justice to the potential contribution which an appropriately trained psychiatrist, working within a multi-disciplinary team, can make towards improving the quality of life for individual patients and also towards optimum functioning of the team itself.

The disadvantages of *not* having designated sessions from a named psychiatrist may usefully be highlighted when presenting a case. Reliance on the local mental health service's sector team or duty rota for occasional referrals is widely perceived as an unsatisfactory system by the various palliative care colleagues from other parts of the country with whom I have discussed this issue. Some have reported being unable to get a psychiatric opinion at all within the requisite timeframe, and others have received opinions which were not helpful. Examples include the diagnosis of 'conversion hysteria' for a patient whose inability to walk was due to a pathological fracture of the femur, or statements such as "he's bound to be depressed if he knows he's dying". Psychiatric support to a palliative care unit is best provided by a named person, preferably a consultant, who can offer experience and continuity.

The job does not require a full-time psychiatrist; two sessions per week is probably sufficient to meet the clinical service requirements for an average-sized palliative care unit. However, fixing these sessions to a set day of the week is not really satisfactory, because time is often so short for the patients involved; most in-patient referrals need to be seen within one or two days. Ideally, therefore, palliative care sessions should be linked with others in a way which permits some flexibility of the working pattern from one week to the next. In my own post this has been satisfactorily accomplished through a link with the Cancer Clinical Centre, of which the palliative care unit is a part; this facilitates early referral, and better continuity of care for patients throughout their 'cancer journey'. This particular post includes four sessions in palliative care, giving opportunities for other activities besides seeing referred patients: teaching and training, involvement with management of the unit, and membership of regional and national bodies for planning palliative care services. It is unlikely that palliative care units outside major teaching centres could support as many as four sessions.

The substantive employment of dedicated support staff from a mental health background may be difficult to justify, partly because the volume of clinical work is not large, and partly because of the high level of psychosocial skills already present within the palliative care team. However, the availability of a psychologist or a clinical nurse specialist in mental health is a great asset and, again, this might be arranged through flexible linkage of the palliative care sessions with other part-time work. Failing this, arrangements might be made to purchase the service on a per-case consultation basis, preferably from a named individual. As mentioned above, in the section on training, the part-time attachment of a junior psychiatrist can be most valuable, both as experience for the trainee and a source of fresh ideas for the consultant. There is also a steady demand from psychiatrists, psychologists and others, often from abroad, seeking training or research placements in palliative care. Each request must be considered on individual merit, but, with some striking exceptions, these attachments cannot be relied upon to maintain the clinical service. All of these possible arrangements demand the careful selection and induction of personnel, because of the importance which attaches to the personalities and attitudes of staff working in palliative care.

My own post is funded and managed from within the general hospital trust, rather than the mental health trust. This helps to simplify day-to-day administration and to identify the psychiatrist as an integral member of the medical team. As regards funding for new posts in other areas, charitable sources should be considered, because these are a mainstay in the development of palliative care services. Individual local charities support specific units; the main national charities are Cancer Relief Macmillan Fund, Marie Curie Cancer Care and the Sue Ryder Foundation (Hospice Information Service, 1996).

References

ADDINGTON-HALL, J. M., MACDONALD, L. D., ANDERSON, H. R., *et al* (1992) Randomised controlled trial of coordinating care for terminally ill cancer patients. *British Medical Journal*, **305**, 1317–1322.
BILLINGS, J. A. & BLOCK, S. (1995) Palliative medicine update: depression. *Journal of Palliative Care*, **11**, 48–54.

BREITBART, W., BRUERA, E., CHOCHINOV, H., *et al* (1995) Neuropsychiatric syndromes and psychological symptoms in patients with advanced cancer. *Journal of Pain and Symptom Management*, **10**, 131–141.

CASSIDY, S. (1986) Emotional distress in terminal cancer. *Journal of the Royal Society of Medicine*, **79**, 717–720.

CHIEF MEDICAL OFFICER'S EXPERT ADVISORY GROUP ON CANCERS (1995) *A Policy Framework for Commissioning Cancer Services*. London: Department of Health.

CHOCHINOV, H. M., WILSON, K. G., ENNS, M., *et al* (1994) Prevalence of depression in the terminally ill: effects of diagnostic criteria and symptom threshold judgments. *American Journal of Psychiatry*, **151**, 537–540.

DRUSS, R. (1995) *The Psychology of Illness: In Sickness and in Health*. Washington, DC: American Psychiatric Press.

GREER, S. & MOOREY, S. (1997) Adjuvant psychological therapy for cancer patients. *Palliative Medicine*, **11**, 240–244.

HARRIS, E. C. & BARRACLOUGH, B. M. (1994) Suicide as an outcome for medical disorders. *Medicine*, **73**, 281–298.

HINTON, J. (1972) Psychiatric consultation in fatal illness. *Proceedings of the Royal Society of Medicine*, **65**, 1035–1038.

HOSPICE INFORMATION SERVICE (1996) *Directory of Hospice and Specialist Palliative Care Services in the United Kingdom and Republic of Ireland*. Available from: Hospice Information Service, St Christopher's Hospice, London.

KEARNEY, M. (1996) *Mortally Wounded*. Dublin: Marino.

KUBLER-ROSS, E. (1970) *On Death and Dying*. London: Tavistock/Routledge.

LICHTER, I. (1991) Some psychological causes of distress in the terminally ill. *Palliative Medicine*, **5**, 138–146.

NATIONAL COUNCIL FOR HOSPICE AND SPECIALIST PALLIATIVE CARE (1995) *Outcome Measures in Palliative Care*. Available from the National Council, 59 Bryanston Street, London W1A 2AZ.

—— (1997) *Feeling Better: Psychosocial Care in Specialist Palliative Care*. Available from the National Council, 59 Bryanston Street, London W1A 2AZ.

NOBLE, T. W. (1996) *Psychological Distress and Symptom Control in Patients with Advanced Cancer: The Effect of Some Simple Interventions*. MD Thesis, University of Sheffield.

PARKES, C. M. (1972) *Bereavement: Studies of Grief in Adult Life*. London: Penguin Books.

POWER, D., KELLY, S., GILSENAN, J., *et al* (1993) Suitable screening tests for cognitive impairment and depression in the terminally ill – a prospective prevalence study. *Palliative Medicine*, **7**, 213–218.

RAMSAY, N. (1992) Referral to a liaison psychiatrist from a palliative care unit. *Palliative Medicine*, **6**, 54–60.

STEDEFORD, A. (1994) *Facing Death* (2nd edn). Oxford: Sobell House Publications.

—— & BLOCH, S. (1979) The psychiatrist in the terminal care unit. *British Journal of Psychiatry*, **135**, 1–6.

TWYCROSS, R. G. (1999) *Introducing Palliative Care* (3rd edn). Oxford: Radcliffe Medical Press.

WOOD, B. C. & MYNORS-WALLIS, L. M. (1997) Problem-solving in palliative care. *Palliative Medicine*, **11**, 49–54.

ZIGMOND, A. S. & SNAITH, R. P. (1983) The Hospital Anxiety and Depression Scale. *Acta Psychiatrica Scandinavica*, **67**, 361–370.

15 Mental health of the National Health Service medical workforce

ANDREW HODGKISS and AMANDA RAMIREZ

The poor mental health of doctors has long been a taboo. It has often been discussed in coded terms, such as 'low morale', and the effects of poor mental health concealed as 'career changes' or early retirement. The stigma of a psychiatric diagnosis within the medical profession makes it difficult to obtain appropriate treatment and to retain employment after recovery unless the illness is concealed. Currently, more open concern about the mental health of doctors and the weaknesses of existing services for those who are sick has been expressed. This is in the context of increasing public awareness of the fallibilty of doctors generally, based on the Bristol Inquiry, the Shipman Case and numerous other incidents. This chapter describes the epidemiology of mental health problems in the medical profession. An overview of the present system of service provision for sick doctors follows, and a consideration of ways of improving those services. Finally, approaches to preventing poor mental health among doctors are examined. Liaison psychiatrists are involved in this work because of their availability within acute trust and their expertise in the common mental health problems experienced by doctors. The suggestions for what a planned, specialist service for doctors might involve are based on the current role and regulation of the medical profession. These aspects of medical life are, however, undergoing considerable change.

Mental health needs of doctors

While doctors enjoy better physical health, they suffer poorer mental health than the general population (British Medical Association, 1992,

1993). In the UK, the suicide rate for medical practitioners is approximately twice the national average (Charlton *et al*, 1993). The prevalence of mental health problems among doctors does not appear to diminish with seniority – high levels of psychiatric morbidity have been reported among senior doctors, including hospital consultants and general practitioners (Caplan, 1994; Blenkin *et al*, 1995; Borrill *et al*, 1996; Ramirez *et al*, 1996). Combining the results of three recent large UK studies, each of which used the General Health Questionnaire, the estimated prevalence of psychiatric morbidity among hospital consultants is 28% (Blenkin *et al*, 1995; Borrill *et al*, 1996; Ramirez *et al*, 1996). This level is similar to the level of about 30% reported among British junior doctors during their pre-registration year (Firth-Cozens, 1987; Borrill *et al*, 1996) and of 29% reported among British medical students (Firth, 1986), using the same assessment approach.

Because their work involves dealing with other people's physical, psychological and social problems, doctors have been considered to be at particular risk of burnout, a specific work-related form of distress (Freudenberger, 1974). Burnout is a syndrome which has no agreed definition, but the components are generally accepted to be emotional exhaustion, treating people in an unfeeling way (depersonalisation) and a sense of low personal accomplishment (Mayou, 1987). Unfortunately, there are no adequate data to compare levels of burnout across doctors of differing seniority or between doctors and other professional groups. Using the Maslach Burnout Inventory, a standardised measure of burnout, the prevalence of these three components has been examined among UK hospital consultants (Ramirez *et al*, 1996) and it appears to be broadly similar to the published norms for American doctors and nurses (Maslach & Jackson, 1996).

It remains uncertain whether burnout exists as a syndrome separate from other negative affective states experienced more pervasively across other domains of life (i.e. psychiatric morbidity), although evidence for its specificity is accruing. For example, while hospital consultants and palliative care physicians report similar levels of psychiatric morbidity, hospital consultants experience higher levels of burnout than their colleagues dedicated to the care of the dying, the majority of whom are based not in hospitals but in hospices (Graham *et al*, 1996).

Overall, there is little evidence that doctors drink more than some other professional groups (Clare, 1990). Medical students consume similar amounts of alcohol as other students, but the overall consumption rate for students is high. Equally, doctors drink no more than others in social class I, but, again, the consumption of alcohol among some other professional groups in social class I, in particular the legal profession, is high.

Data on the use of drugs among doctors is sparse, particularly within the UK. A small American study showed that doctors used mood-altering drugs, such as stimulants, tranquillisers and sedatives, more than other college graduates (Vaillant *et al*, 1970). Unsurprisingly, there is little information on the use of non-prescription and controlled drugs, and it is difficult to know if doctors use such drugs more than others. Doctors' misuse of drugs is likely, at least in part, to be a reflection of their availability, as well as an indication of poor mental health.

Risk factors for poor mental health among doctors

The stresses inherent in the practice of medicine appear to precipitate burnout and psychiatric morbidity in those who are psychologically vulnerable. The occupational risk factors and the predisposing socio-demographic and personal risk factors are summarised in Table 15.1 (Firth-Cozens, 1987; Cooper *et al*, 1989; Borrill *et al*, 1996; Ramirez *et al*, 1996).

One of the main occupational risk factors for poor mental health among doctors is, of course, high levels of stress at work. The predominant source of job stress for doctors in all specialities and at all levels of seniority is overload and its effect on home life. For

TABLE 15.1
Risk factors for poor mental health among doctors

Occupational factors	Socio-demographic and personal factors
High levels of job stress from: Overload and its effect on home life Organisational constraints (e.g. feeling poorly managed and resourced) Dealing with patients' suffering	Being female Being single[1] Young age[1] Fewer years in the job[1] Other stressful life events Family psychiatric history
Low levels of job satisfaction from: Having good relationships with patients, relatives and staff Having professional status and esteem Feeling well managed and resourced Deriving intellectual stimulation Having variety in the job[1] Having a high level of autonomy[1]	Childhood experience of illness, death and emotional neglect Particular personality traits (e.g. obsessive–compulsive traits)
Inadequate training in communication and management skills	

1. Based on evidence related to senior doctors only.

consultants, at least, job satisfaction has been shown to protect their mental health against the adverse effects of job stress (Ramirez *et al*, 1996). Job satisfaction among senior doctors working both in the hospital and in primary care is related to the amount of responsibility given, the freedom to choose working methods and the amount of variety in the job. Faced with the high demands of medicine, the degree of autonomy senior doctors have over their work is an important determinant of mental health.

A further major source of job stress for doctors is difficulties they experience in communicating with patients and relatives. Particularly stressful scenarios include breaking bad news, and dealing with distressed, angry or complaining patients and relatives. These difficulties predominate for junior house officers (Firth-Cozens, 1987) and senior house officers (Williams *et al*, 1997), general practitioners (Cooper *et al*, 1989) and hospital consultants (Ramirez *et al*, 1996). Feeling insufficiently trained in communication skills is associated with an increased risk of burnout among senior clinicians. A similar increased risk has been described among those senior clinicians who feel insufficiently trained in management skills (Ramirez *et al*, 1996).

Gender has a marked influence on the mental health of hospital doctors. Female doctors have been shown to experience a significantly higher prevalence of psychiatric morbidity than their male counterparts (37% versus 23% for consultants and 41% versus 26% for junior doctors) (Borrill *et al*, 1996). This striking gender difference also applies to hospital managers and cannot be explained by gender differences in work-related factors such as perceived work demands and patient contact. This gender difference is not evident among other staff in National Health Service (NHS) trusts, such as nurses, radiographers, technical/laboratory staff and clerical staff. It seems, therefore, that it is not being female *per se* which is a risk factor, but being female in particular jobs, namely medicine and management, where the NHS culture and hierarchies may have a more adverse impact on women than men (Borrill *et al*, 1996). Interestingly, in general practice women seem to enjoy better health compared with normative groups, while men experience more anxiety than the norms (Cooper *et al*, 1989).

Rates of burnout, but not psychiatric morbidity, appear to differ across consultants working in different specialities (Blenkin *et al*, 1995; Ramirez *et al*, 1996). For example, radiologists suffer higher levels of burnout than surgeons, gastroenterologists and oncologists (Ramirez *et al*, 1996). To what extent such a difference in risk across specialities reflects differences in the nature of the work or differences in the nature of the doctor is difficult to discern, although it seems likely that the particular personal characteristics of doctors attracted into different specialist careers determine their degree of psychological vulnerability. Psychiatrists have been shown to differ from surgeons and physicians by having higher levels of neuroticism, openness and agreeableness, but lower levels of conscientiousness. While psychiatrists report significantly fewer clinical work demands than their surgical and medical colleagues, they report significantly more burnout and depression (Deary *et al*, 1996).

Reluctance of doctors to seek help

A corollary of the necessary preoccupation with the needs of patients is a reluctance among doctors to admit that they themselves can become patients. Instead, there is a tendency to deny health problems, to continue to work when ill and to believe that ill health, especially the inability to cope with stress, is stigmatising. These attitudes are fostered in medical training, where students learn that feeling distressed is perceived as weakness and the expectation is that you 'tough it through' any illness. Related to this is a reluctance to 'inform' on colleagues who are clearly neglecting mental health problems, out of a sense of professional loyalty. Doctors notoriously rely on self-medication and, where they recognise the need for advice, direct self-referral to hospital consultants and 'corridor' consultations with colleagues. As a consequence there is little formally recorded evidence of their mental ill health and the culture of non-recognition of mental health problems is reinforced.

These attitudes naturally predispose doctors to be ill-informed about, or at least suspicious of, the nature and possible effectiveness of services designed specifically to address their mental health problems. Such lack of knowledge reinforces the culture of denial, it being easier to ignore a problem if there are no obvious and reliable means available to provide a solution. This situation is compounded by the widespread distrust doctors have regarding the confidentiality of available services. The tendency is for the support services to be called upon only when problems created by a doctor's poor mental health have become crises or are obviously endangering patients.

Mentally ill doctors as a special case?

Doctors with poor mental health can generate complex problems, the handling of which may pose enormous challenges. There is a case, albeit a controversial one, for viewing the mental health problems of doctors as different from those of other NHS staff. Doctors are expensive to train and to pay, while their clinical decisions account for a large part of NHS expenditure. Moreover, their mental health is vital to the safety and quality of patients' care.

There are multiple issues to consider in relation to a mentally ill doctor, including the need to protect patients, the duty of other doctors to report problems, concern to ensure that colleagues are supported, helped and enabled to continue to fulfil the roles for which they were trained, and the responsibility of a good employer to care for its staff. Strongly held and polarised views often exist among doctors, nursing staff and managers.

Current service provision for doctors with mental health problems

The main way of helping doctors with mental health problems is through a series of national procedural frameworks and local health services. There are acknowledged weaknesses in these procedures and services, which are patchy and not well known or understood. Four important reports have been published by the Nuffield Provincial Hospitals Trust describing current service provision, attitudes within the medical profession to these services and pathways to care for sick doctors, and making some recommendations for change (Silvester *et al*, 1994; McKevitt *et al*, 1995, 1996; Nuffield Provincial Hospitals Trust Working Party, 1996). Broadly, there are four types of service provision, and these are discussed under separate headings, below.

Statutory provision

The primary concern of the statutory services is to prevent harm to patients. They include the Health Committee of the General Medical Council (GMC), the hospital-based 'three wise men' procedure and a similar mechanism based on local medical committees for general practitioners. Doctors are generally referred to them by colleagues acting on their ethical obligation to report.

Practically all cases referred to the GMC's health procedures involve alcohol, drugs or mental illness. The health procedures are designed not only to protect patients but also to rehabilitate sick doctors. They may involve four main stages: preliminary consideration of the evidence, medical examination of the sick doctor, medical supervision and rehabilitation of the sick doctor, and referral to the Health Committee, which has the power to suspend doctors. Involvement of système

the GMC has the drawback that it is defined by statute and, strictly speaking, currently limited to the professional conduct of doctors who are severely impaired. Only now is the GMC introducing a system for dealing with poorly performing doctors. Moreover, some doctors are intimidated by the GMC's disciplinary connotations and fear that, if they refer a colleague to it, it will endanger their colleague's livelihood. As a consequence, such referrals are very few: about 37 per year.

The 'three wise men' procedure, in which a panel of consultants in a hospital has the power to intervene when patients are at risk of harm because of a doctor's illness, is often criticised as ineffective and is not widely understood. This criticism is partially justified, as the effectiveness of the procedure has, to a great extent, been compromised by the secrecy and confidentiality which characterises it. However, there are numerous examples of mentally ill doctors who have been identified by it, treated and successfully returned to work without anyone in the hospital being aware of the problem. The same is true of the work of members of local medical committees on behalf of mentally ill general practitioners.

Employer provision

All NHS authorities and trusts have a responsibility to ensure that their staff have access to confidential occupational health services. Although these services are potentially a valuable source of support to stressed and mentally ill doctors, doctors in general have not regarded them in this light. This is related to the dual function of the occupational health service as adviser to the employer as well as advocate of the employee. Occupational health physicians have a remit to provide information to the employer about the doctor-patient's fitness to work, but not clinical details. They will not breach confidentiality to the employer without signed consent. They also have a wider remit to provide information for selection procedures, to undertake routine medical examinations and to ensure health and safety at work. Currently, occupational health services exist in only skeletal form in the NHS and make little or no provision for general practitioners. It is not clear that occupational physicians have the necessary skills to deal with the mental health problems common among doctors, although they can be effective in referring doctor-patients appropriately and supporting their return to work.

Independent and self-help agencies

These include the National Counselling Service for Sick Doctors (NCSSD), the British Doctors and Dentists Group (assisting with alcohol and drug problems), the Association of Anaesthetists' Sick Doctors Scheme, the British Medical Association's telephone counselling service and the Doctors' Support Network. The NCSSD, which was set up in 1985, aims to provide an accessible, confidential and non-coercive counselling service to doctors. Doctors in need of help are linked up to a local adviser, who provides assistance in seeking help. Psychiatrists from a list maintained by the Royal College of Psychiatrists are available to provide appropriate management. Unfortunately, the NCSSD is not widely used and its effectiveness has not yet been reported on.

The British Medical Association's recently established confidential national telephone counselling service received over 3300 calls from doctors, medical students and their families during its first year of operation. Fifty-seven per cent of the calls were from women, despite the fact that they make up less than one-third of all doctors in Britain. Thirty-six per cent of calls dealt with emotional problems, particularly stress, anxiety and depression.

Local mental health service provision

Much of the direct clinical care of mentally ill doctors falls to local psychiatric colleagues. Currently, it is unusual for there to be contractual arrangements for this activity; rather, it is still done on a 'grace and favour' basis. Hospital doctors may be seen by a psychiatric colleague working in the same trust. Some enlightened trusts have made reciprocal arrangements with other trusts, so that doctors can be seen by a psychiatrist in another trust in order to maintain confidentiality. As general psychiatrists re-deploy from the acute general hospital to the community and focus ever more on severe mental illness, it falls increasingly to the liaison and academic psychiatrists remaining in hospitals to look after mentally ill doctors.

Assessing and treating doctors with mental health problems

Assessing and treating doctors with mental health problems raises particular issues for the psychiatrist. The standard of care expected by mentally ill doctors is high. In effect, they need to be accorded 'privileged patient status', equivalent to that of a private patient. This is in part because of the need to maintain confidentiality with respect to other NHS personnel. Their care is usually provided by the consultant *alone*. This work is often done out of hours, not only to maintain confidentiality but also because there is no other available time (for the psychiatrist or the doctor-patient). Thus the management of doctors with mental health problems makes disproportionate demands on the consultant psychiatrist compared with other NHS patients. There is very little documentation of the level of NHS psychiatric activity incurred by doctor-patients.

Not surprisingly, a proportion of doctors with mental health problems seek care within the private sector, where confidentiality can be more assured and they can be guaranteed consultant-only care in comfortable facilities. The numbers of doctors seeking private help is, of course, unknown, but it is evident that the private hospitals are responding to the market of mentally ill doctors, particularly those who misuse alcohol and drugs.

Referral of doctor-patients is often late and via an unorthodox route. The psychiatrist must set aside any sense of irritation about this. The shared background between treating doctor and doctor-patient ought to be an aid to empathy, yet identification with a mentally ill doctor can provoke anxiety since it threatens any fantasies of invulnerability the psychiatrist harbours. Seeing doctors reminds us of the deficiencies of the physical environment in which we work and the untherapeutic in-patient environment that is commonplace on many overstretched acute psychiatric wards.

Before embarking on any assessment interview, an explicit discussion of confidentiality and its limits is useful. The details of what will be told to whom and why need to be negotiated. As a way of building trust and avoiding later recriminations, the doctor-patient can be invited to see the assessment letter before dispatch to the referrer or general practitioner. If confidence must be breached at some point to protect the public, it is good practice to tell the doctor-patient that this is planned and why it is regarded as essential.

During the assessment interview eliciting, exploring and respecting the health beliefs and treatment preferences of the patient are particularly important. Most doctors are intelligent and opinionated. It can be tempting to collude in self-management in the hope of somehow lessening one's own clinical responsibility. This is a disservice to such patients, who should be relieved of the burden of deciding their own care. Another area to be included in the assessment is the patient's view of the impact of the illness on work. This can be a useful marker of insight, particularly when an informant history from a colleague or manager is available for comparison, and is relevant to decisions about fitness to practise.

Admitting doctors to acute psychiatric wards can be problematic and is becoming increasingly untenable. Elizabeth Armstrong, of the Doctors' Support Network, recently recounted this story:

"One doctor, suffering suicidal depression, was repeatedly asked
by ward staff, who knew he was a doctor, to check ward drugs and
prescriptions. Furthermore, once fellow patients realised he was a
doctor, they also consulted him." (Armstrong, 1997)

When selecting treatments for sick doctors, consideration needs
to be given to the longer term. Non-sedative antidepressants should
be chosen whenever possible so that return to work on continuation
therapy or long-term prophylaxis is possible. Long-term psychotherapy is likely to be unsuitable for a junior doctor who will be
moving around the country over the next year or two.

Doctors who misuse drugs and alcohol present special problems.
Ghodse (1995) has described clinical management approaches to
substance-misusing doctors. He suggests that two doctors, one a
colleague in a supportive capacity and one with an interest in
substance misuse, confront the doctor-patient with a prearranged
treatment offer. Confronting the issue without an action plan can
cause despair. Failure of the doctor to respond to such persuasion
should trigger a referral to the GMC Health Committee.

Often substance misuse affects doctors' behaviour rather than their
competence itself. Difficult judgements have to be made about how
much their behaviour affects patient care, professional relationships
and teamwork. Here the opportunities for stigma and hostile attitudes
are particularly great, and decisions about how and when to treat,
as well as whether the doctor should remain at work, are particularly
important.

Impact of NHS reforms on existing services

The existing provision for mentally ill doctors is inadequate and is
threatened by aspects of recent structural changes in the NHS. In
particular, the traditional pattern of providing out-of-district
psychiatric care has been threatened by limited budgets and contracts.

The dissolution of the regional level of management has reduced
the scope for the informal resolution of problems through the 'three
wise men' mechanism, including arranging for the temporary removal
from duty of a doctor who had become unfit to practise, for treatment
on sick leave, drawing on the assistance of the district and regional
medical officers, and using, if necessary, the resource of super-
numerary posts controlled by the latter. It is increasingly clear that
the support for an individual doctor in difficulty will largely be a
matter for the employing trust.

The role of the clinical director in the handling of sick doctors is
unclear. Through audit and managerial scrutiny they should be

among the first to know about under-performing clinicians, yet there are doubts as to how they might respond. If a clinical director realises that a doctor is under-performing for reasons of poor mental health, there is a need to address the personal problem for the doctor, the issue of patient safety and issues of cost and directorate performance standards. These may create tensions and conflicts of interest and loyalty, which may work against a more sympathetic, informal approach to the problems of the doctor concerned. Some trusts are now keen contractually to oblige senior doctors to 'whistle blow' on sick or incompetent colleagues, having wearied at the sluggish response to the longstanding ethical obligation to do so. Whether concern and care or discipline and dismissal would follow remains to be seen.

Development of better services for doctors with mental health problems

The principles that need to be observed in developing better services for doctors with mental health problems include:

(a) ensuring the safety of patients;
(b) ensuring optimal care for the doctor-patient;
(c) protecting the longer-term employment prospects of the doctor-patient – for the benefit of the doctor-patient and the NHS.

For these principles to be implemented, both local and more overarching regional and national initiatives are required to define and implement policies related to

(a) the identification of doctors with mental health problems;
(b) their assessment;
(c) their treatment;
(d) the reporting and monitoring of cases.

At a local acute trust level, the group responsible for developing such policies would appropriately include the medical director, the occupational physician, the chair of the 'three wise men' procedure and an interested psychiatrist. Where there are liaison psychiatrists, then the task is likely to fall to them. This is because, compared with their colleagues in general psychiatry, they are more available and accessible to the acute trust. Also, by the nature of the rest of their work in the general hospital, liaison psychiatrists have particular expertise in the common mental health problems that doctors experience.

At a regional level, a framework is required to facilitate the implementation of local policy. The Working Party established by the Nuffield Provincial Hospitals Trust under the chairmanship of Sir Maurice Shock (Nuffield Provincial Hospitals Trust Working Party, 1996) recommended that a network of independent regional bodies be established devoted to reviewing and reporting on services to sick doctors. It is through such regional bodies that reciprocal arrangements between trusts, intended to maintain confidentiality, could be organised. The Working Party proposed that an individual senior doctor should be identified in each locality to act as a first point of contact for those in need, or those reporting illness in others, and to arrange further care. This might be the liaison psychiatrist, who would be available either to doctors in the trust or to those from another trust, depending on whether reciprocal arrangements had been made. The current 'grace and favour' system under which psychiatrists provide care for doctor-patients would need to be abandoned. In recognition of the time-consuming nature of this work, it would require a dedicated and acknowledged sessional commitment. The Working Party recommended improvements in locum cover for short-term sick leave, increased levels of general practitioner registration among doctors and funding for extra-contractual referrals when required.

Specific issues that will need to be considered are discussed below.

Identification

Some doctors will recognise that they have a mental health problem and will seek advice and care from their general practitioner, a national service (e.g. the British Medical Association's telephone counselling service) or a psychiatric colleague. It might be anticipated that these doctor-patients will have mental health problems at the less severe end of the spectrum. Of more concern are those doctors who do not self-refer. They will be identified by colleagues and should be referred to the nominated psychiatrist in the interest of the doctor-patient's mental health and also to the clinical director if there are concerns about conduct and performance that may jeopardise patient safety.

Assessment

Assessment services may either be provided within the trust in which a doctor-patient works or elsewhere through a reciprocal arrangement. The assessment needs to be conducted by a skilled psychiatrist and should include an assessment of risk to patients as well as the needs of the doctor-patient. Assessment *per se* is unlikely to result in large costs to any one provider unit.

Treatment

Treatment should ideally be provided outside the trust in which the doctor works, for example by reciprocal arrangement within the NHS or by arrangement with a private provider. The issue of who pays for these services, particularly aspects which are expensive, especially long-term in-patient care, need to be considered. Trusts are unlikely to be prepared to pay for this. Arrangements are needed with the health authority in which the doctor-patient resides.

Reporting and monitoring

Mechanisms need to be established whereby issues regarding fitness to work are fed back from the assessing/treating service to the occupational health service of the doctor-patient's employing trust and thence to the clinical director. Equally, mechanisms need to be in place to monitor the doctor-patient's competence, if that has been compromised by the mental health problems.

Primary care trusts need to adopt a similar approach to service provision for general practitioners with mental health problems.

Prevention

In addition to improving the system for detecting, managing and sometimes removing doctors with mental health problems, there needs to be a focus on preventing those problems (Smith, 1997). This should include helping the public and medical school applicants to understand better the limitations of medicine, as such action should reduce the pressure on doctors. Those seeking a career in medicine who are vulnerable should not be denied entry, but should be given greater support from the beginning. The prevailing medical culture that encourages doctors to hide their difficulties and distress needs to shift to one which engenders more self-awareness and self-care, as well as facilitating the sharing of problems and seeking appropriate help. This may well happen anyway as medicine becomes less male dominated. Healthier work patterns need to be developed, with shorter hours, better training to increase the doctors' personal competence in meeting the demands of contemporary medicine, better appraisal and guidance, and more flexibility.

Conclusions

There has been growing recent concern about the levels of psychiatric morbidity among doctors and a substantial research literature quantifying this has appeared in the last decade. Suicide and mood disorders are definitely overrepresented in this professional group. It is clear that self-regulation of the medical profession with respect to sick doctors is now under intense scrutiny from both NHS managers and the public. Insisting on the adequacy of current arrangements for the detection and management of doctors with mental health problems is not an option, least of all since traditional responses, such as out-of-district care, have been disrupted by NHS changes. New initiatives are needed and if the medical profession, notably psychiatrists, do not devise these, health authorities and hospital trust managers will.

Some consideration of the care of doctor-patients with mental health problems should be included in the training of psychiatrists, and the particular mental health needs of women in medicine require examination. The poor mental health of doctors harms not only themselves but also their patients. Developing better systems for detecting, managing and also preventing such problems will help both doctors and patients.

Acknowledgements

We are grateful to Professor Michael Richards, Dr Elspeth Guthrie and Dr David Snashall for their comments on the typescript.

References

ARMSTRONG, E. (1997) Rehabilitating troubled doctors. *British Medical Journal Classified*, **314**, 2–3.

BLENKIN, H., DEARY, I., SADLER, A., *et al* (1995) Stress in NHS consultants. *British Medical Journal*, **310**, 534.

BORRILL, C., WALL, T., WEST, M., *et al* (1996) *Mental Health of the Workforce in NHS Trusts*. Institute of Work Psychology, University of Sheffield, and Department of Psychology, University of Leeds.

BRITISH MEDICAL ASSOCIATION (1992) *Stress and the Medical Profession*. London: BMA.

—— (1993) *The Morbidity and Mortality of the Medical Profession*. London: British Medical Association Board of Science and Education.

CAPLAN, R. (1994) Stress, anxiety and depression in hospital consultants, general practitioners and senior health managers. *British Medical Journal*, **309**, 1261–1263.

CHARLTON, J., KELLY, S., DUNNELL, K., *et al* (1993) Suicide deaths in England and Wales: trends in factors associated with suicide deaths. *Popular Trends*, **69**, 34–42.

CLARE, A. (1990) The alcohol problem in universities and the professions. *Alcohol and Alcoholism*, **25**, 277–285.

COOPER, C., ROUT, U. & FARAGHER, B. (1989) Mental health, job satisfaction, and job stress among general practitioners. *British Medical Journal*, **298**, 366–370.

DEARY, I., AGIUS, R. & SADLER, A (1996) Personality and stress in consultant psychiatrists. *International Journal of Social Psychology*, **42**, 112–123.

FIRTH, J. (1986) Levels and sources of stress in medical students. *British Medical Journal*, **292**, 1177–1180.

FIRTH-COZENS, J. (1987) Emotional distress in junior house officers. *British Medical Journal*, **295**, 533–536.

FREUDENBERGER, H. (1974). Staff burnout. *Journal of Social Issues*, **30**, 159–165.

GHODSE, H. (1995) *Drugs and Addictive Behaviour: A Guide to Treatment*, pp. 277–280. London: Blackwell Scientific.

GRAHAM, J., RAMIREZ, A., CULL, A., *et al* (1996) Job stress and satisfaction among palliative physicians. *Palliative Medicine*, **10**, 185–194.

MASLACH, C. & JACKSON, S. (1996) *Maslach Burnout Inventory*. Palo Alto: Consulting Psychologists' Press.

MAYOU, R. (1987) Burnout. *British Medical Journal*, **295**, 284–285.

McKEVITT, C., MORGAN, M., SIMPSON, J., *et al* (1995) *Doctors' Health and Needs for Service*. London: Nuffield Provincial Hospitals Trust.

——, —— & HOLLAND, W. (1996) *Protecting and Promoting Doctors' Health: The Work Environment and Counselling Services in Three Sites*. London: Nuffield Provincial Hospitals Trust.

NUFFIELD PROVINCIAL HOSPITALS TRUST WORKING PARTY (1996) *Taking Care of Doctors' Health. Reducing Avoidable Stress and Improving Services for Doctors Who Fall Ill*. London: Nuffield Provincial Hospitals Trust.

RAMIREZ, A., GRAHAM, J., RICHARDS, M., *et al* (1996) Mental health of hospital consultants: the effects of stress and satisfaction at work. *Lancet*, **347**, 724–728.

SILVESTER, S., ALLEN, H., WITHEY, C., *et al* (1994) *The Provision of Medical Services to Sick Doctors. A Conspiracy of Friendliness?* London: Nuffield Provincial Hospitals Trust.

SMITH, R. (1997) All doctors are problem doctors. *British Medical Journal*, **314**, 841–842.

VAILLANT, G., BRIGHTON, J. & MCARTHUR, C. (1970) Physicians' use of mood altering drugs. A 20 year follow-up report. *New England Journal of Medicine*, **282**, 365–370.

WILLIAMS, S., DALE, J., GLUCKMAN, E., *et al* (1997) Senior house officers' work-related stressors, psychological distress and confidence in performing clinical tasks in accident and emergency: a questionnaire study. *British Medical Journal*, **314**, 713–718.

16 Joint working with physicians and surgeons

MICHAEL SHARPE, DAVID PROTHEROE and ALLAN HOUSE

Need for joint working

Human illnesses are conventionally considered as *either* bodily *or* mental in nature (Kirmayer, 1988). One practical consequence of this dualistic thinking is that hospital services have been developed accordingly; there are medical/surgical services for patients with bodily illness and psychiatric/psychological services for those with mental ailments. Consequently, the psychological and psychiatric care of patients attending medical and surgical services tends to be neglected. While this neglect is potentially undesirable for all patients, it becomes particularly problematic for those patients whose problems have a substantial psychiatric or psychological component.

These 'psychiatric' aspects of patients' illnesses are clinically significant and are associated with:

(a) a worse outcome from medical treatment (Mayou & Sharpe, 1995);
(b) increased utilisation of medical care and hence medical costs (House, 1995);
(c) physician frustration (Lin *et al*, 1991).

Common examples of problems with a substantial psychiatric or psychological component are given below.

Patients with somatic symptoms that are unexplained by a medical condition

Somatic complaints for which the assessing physician can find no clear biomedical explanation, sometimes called somatisation symptoms, are common in patients attending medical services (Mayou *et al*, 1995). For example, one study found that such complaints constituted a third of 343 new out-patients at a general hospital (Hamilton *et al*, 1996). Such symptoms also account for a substantial minority of hospital admissions (Fink, 1992).

Patients with depression and anxiety in addition to their medical condition

Emotional disorders frequently accompany medical conditions. The emotional disorder is then referred to as being comorbid. Comorbid depression or anxiety is found in 10–50% of medical patients (Mayou & Sharpe, 1995).

Patients with abnormal illness beliefs and behaviours

Patients' beliefs about their illness may differ from their doctors' (Sharpe *et al*, 1994). For example, they may *fear* that they have a serious medical condition requiring medical treatment when their doctor does not, as in anxious hypochondriasis (Barsky, 1983). They may *believe* that their symptoms are due to a medical condition when their doctor does not, as with patients who have strong convictions about what pathology underlies their symptoms in chronic fatigue syndrome (Schweitzer *et al*, 1994). These illness beliefs may lead to conflict in the doctor–patient relationship (Sharpe *et al*, 1994), may complicate management and lead to a poorer outcome for the patient.

Patients with behavioural problems such as substance misuse and self-harm

Unhelpful coping behaviours, such as taking excess alcohol, may complicate or even cause medical conditions. Problem drinking has been found in a substantial proportion of medical out-patients (Persson & Magnusson, 1987). Alcohol withdrawal is a major cause of delirium in medical and surgical patients. Deliberate self-harm, usually by overdose, is a major cause of medical admission and carries a risk of subsequent suicide (Hawton, 1996).

Patients with acute or chronic cognitive impairment

Cognitive impairment may be acute (delirium) or chronic (dementia). In either case it is associated with management difficulties due to behavioural problems, with poor treatment adherence and increased mortality.

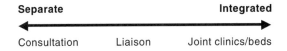

Fig. 16.1. Psychiatric services to medical patients – a spectrum of integration.

Psychiatric/psychological services

From the above it follows that there is a powerful argument for improving the psychiatric and psychological management of patients attending medical and surgical services. This requires some violation of the medical/surgical and psychiatric/psychological divide. There are a number of ways of doing this. These can be portrayed on a continuum that ranges from simply providing a free-standing psychiatric service within the general hospital, which operates in parallel with the medical and surgical services, to fully integrated joint medical–psychiatric services (Fig. 16.1). These different methods of joint working are examined below. In-patients and out-patients are considered separately, although in practice there may be considerable overlap in the issues and in the services themselves.

In-patients

There are a number of ways of working with physicians and surgeons to provide a psychiatric/psychological service to in-patients on medical and surgical units. Each has advantages and disadvantages.

Specialist psychiatric beds in the general hospital

The development of psychiatric units within general hospitals made psychiatry geographically more accessible to the medical and surgical wards. None the less, the in-patient management of medically ill patients has rarely been feasible in most general hospital psychiatric units, so that the service provided to the general hospital by these units has been restricted to little more than the removal of disturbed patients from the general wards.

Advantages

- Obviates the need for interhospital transfer and allows the physician/surgeon to continue to visit the patient

Disadvantages

- Most patients are psychotic, making the ward an unsuitable environment for the severely physically ill
- Very limited capacity to cope with medical conditions

Consultation to medical and surgical units

The simplest ways of bridging the divide between medical and psychiatric services is for the psychiatrist to leave the psychiatric unit and visit patients on medical or surgical wards. In this style of working, psychiatric staff respond to requests for an opinion, see the patient and then advise general hospital staff on management. Often all communication is by notes and there is no direct contact between doctors. The physician or surgeon remains in overall control of patient management and may or may not implement the psychiatrist's recommendations (Huyse *et al*, 1990). This is probably the most common form of liaison psychiatry service in the UK (Mayou *et al*, 1990).

Advantages

- Simple and cheap
- Deals with high profile problems rapidly

Disadvantages

- Little educational value
- Little effect on medical/surgical practice
- Limited effect on patterns of management
- Risk that the psychiatrist becomes just a 'doctor who takes a history'

Liaison with medical and surgical units

Liaison refers to meeting with the staff of the medical or surgical unit in order to discuss general issues of management as well as individual cases. It is a valuable supplement to consultation and is important in influencing what types of patients are referred for consultation. This form of working is frequently offered on a limited basis to interested units. It requires attendance at regular meetings and is based on the building of working relationships over time.

Advantages

- Allows the shaping of referral patterns
- Provides an opportunity to educate medical staff
- Potentially able to influence the management of more patients

Disadvantages

• Psychiatry still marginal to patients' management
• Nature of contact can degenerate into diffuse discussion or revert to consultation

Joint medical–psychiatric in-patient units

There are several models for jointly managed beds, and below we briefly consider those of the USA, Germany and the UK.

Medical–psychiatric units in the USA

Specialised medical–psychiatric units began to be established in the USA in the late 1970s (Kathol *et al*, 1992). These units admitted and treated patients with combined physical and psychiatric illness. Since their first introduction, a number of different types have been set up, reflecting local staff interests, resources and service needs. Some, such as in-patient units for chronic pain, have developed as a support for a hospital-wide ward consultation service; others, such as those dealing with acute confusion, are part of a liaison service with care shared between named consultants from different specialities.

A survey of 11 units in the USA (Harsch *et al*, 1991) revealed a marked variation in the types of psychiatric and physical problems treated. The commonest psychiatric problems were affective disorder, organic psychiatric syndromes and schizophrenia. Common coexisting physical illnesses included neurological/ central nervous system disease, cardiovascular disease and gastro-intestinal disorders. It is noteworthy that only 27% of the patients in these units were transferred from other specialities in the same hospital. Many patients were admitted from the local community and others were tertiary referrals. All of the units surveyed were able to provide intravenous therapy, oxygen and total general nursing care.

Psychosomatic units in Germany

In-patient units for the treatment of psychosomatic illness are a particular feature of services in Germany. These units treat a different range of illnesses from their North American counterparts. Physical comorbidity is lower and psychosomatic illness is treated with a more psychodynamically influenced approach (Hertzog, 1991).

Joint medical–psychiatric beds in the UK

In the UK, many old-age medical units and some paediatric units enjoy a degree of integration, with joint ward rounds and varying degrees of joint management, but we are not aware of any medical–psychiatric units on the American model (Mayou *et al*, 1990). However, a few pain management services offer a multi-disciplinary in-patient environment, with some similarities to the German psychosomatic clinic – but usually run on cognitive–behavioural rather than on psychodynamic lines (Williams *et al*, 1993).

Advantages

- Optimal way to manage effectively patients with combined severe medical and psychiatric problems

Disadvantages

- Expensive
- Risk becoming a 'dustbin' for the hospital's most difficult patients (borderline personality disorder, dementia), who are also often hard to discharge

In-patient services – conclusions

Most hospitals with liaison psychiatry or psychology services to their in-patient beds have adopted a consultation model, supplemented by varying degrees of liaison. While developments in the USA appear to be currently favouring the setting up of specialist medical–psychiatric units for persons with combinations of severe medical and psychiatric illness, such units have not so far been copied in the UK, probably for reasons of cost. We suggest that an efficient consultation service supplemented by liaison, with as many units as resources will allow, is probably the best current model.

There are strong arguments for a limited number of jointly nursed, jointly managed medical–psychiatric beds in the general hospital for patients who are very sick and not well managed by existing medical or psychiatric services. An example would be the severely ill anorexic patient. However, such beds are likely to be expensive to nurse and demanding on the liaison psychiatrist's time.

Out-patients

Several forms of service have been described (Dolinar, 1993), again each with its own advantages and disadvantages (Sullivan, 1993).

The general psychiatry clinic in the general hospital

In some general hospitals, general psychiatry clinics are held in the general hospital. The reasons for this include a convenient location and an attempt to avoid the stigma of a clinic based in a mental hospital. However, as with in-patient units sited within general hospitals, such clinics frequently take only referrals from outside the hospital and function in isolation form the rest of the organisation.

Advantages
- Gives an opportunity for the psychiatrist to meet medical colleagues

Disadvantages
- Rarely see referrals from the hospital
- Other patients attending make the nature of the clinic clear

A specialist liaison psychiatry out-patient service

This is a common form of liaison psychiatry out-patient service. The medical or surgical services continue unchanged and patients selected by the physician or surgeon may be referred to the specialist service. The liaison psychiatry out-patient clinic is based on the same model as the specialist medical clinics; in this sense, liaison psychiatry becomes another speciality clinic, such as cardiology or orthopaedics. These clinics share the medical out-patient accommodation or more commonly are in another area of the hospital designated as 'psychiatry out-patients'. All that is needed to set up such a service are clinic rooms and the time of a psychiatrist – although the contribution of trainees and a multi-disciplinary treatment team are desirable additions.

Advantages
- Easy to organise and a familiar model, therefore comfortable for psychiatric and psychology staff
- Allows concentration of scarce psychiatric/psychological assessment and treatment resources in one clinic
- Provides a useful forum for teaching medical students and psychiatric trainees

Disadvantages
- Is dependent on the physician or surgeon to identify cases requiring psychiatric care

- Is likely to be stigmatised as 'psychiatric' and therefore to be unpopular with patients and other doctors; consequently, patients may not be referred or may not attend
- There is no real integration with other medical services and the educational value is therefore limited. In particular, there is no real challenge to the dualistic thinking of doctors or patients (i.e. patients continue to be seen as either medical or psychiatric)
- There tends to be a one-way transfer of patients from medicine/surgery to psychiatry/psychology – the result may be a clogging up of the psychiatry service

Providing consultations to out-patients

In this type of service, the standard in-patient consultation model as described above is simply extended to cover out-patients. Thus, if physicians are concerned about a patient attending the medical clinic, they call the liaison psychiatrist and ask for an urgent consultation. If available, the psychiatrist, probably a junior, comes to the clinic and interviews the patient in an available room. The psychiatrist then reports back to the physician. Outcomes include removal of the patient, offering the patient an appointment in the psychiatric clinic and advising the clinician on management.

Advantages

- Requires few resources
- Readily accepted way of working

Disadvantages

- Can handle only a very small number of referrals
- Very limited contact between psychiatry and clinic
- Largely a 'removal' service

Liaison with specific medical or surgical clinics

Having a designated psychiatrist or psychologist form an ongoing liaison with a specific clinic can enhance the consultation model. Psychiatrists may meet regularly with the clinic staff and may make themselves available in the clinic to give advice on management.

Advantages

- Ongoing input to clinic is possible
- Opportunity to educate clinic staff

Disadvantages

- If there is nothing to do, it may be inefficient
- Dependent on clinic staff for referrals
- Limited facilities for offering specific assessments or treatments

An integrated medical–psychiatric clinic

At its simplest, an integrated service means that the psychiatrist or psychologist and physician or surgeon both contribute to the assessment and treatment of a patient at the same time and in cooperation. As anyone who has ever had work done on their house knows, there are practical advantages in being able to coordinate the work of the different trades and potentially dire consequences of their working independently. Thus joint medical–psychiatric working should not only reduce the need for multiple clinic visits but also prevent the equivalent of having the roof replaced only to have the plumber find later that the leak was from the pipes.

For out-patients, integration between medical/surgical and psychiatric/psychological clinics means that patients get a combined assessment from a single referral. Such clinics may also be more acceptable to patients than purely psychiatric ones (Sullivan, 1993). An example of this is a Dutch pelvic pain service described by Peters (Peters *et al*, 1991). Patients were randomised to either a standard gynaecological assessment followed by referral to psychology when investigations were negative or to an integrated medical–psychological assessment and management programme. The latter group was found to have a better outcome one year later. A similar approach to back pain in a German clinic was also found to be successful (Basler *et al*, 1997).

Advantages

- Provides a true 'one-stop' way of addressing the full range of the patient's problems, and therefore should minimise the possibilities of misdiagnosis and mismanagement
- Some evidence it improves patient outcome
- Optimises the opportunities for education for both psychiatrist and physician and is an ideal opportunity to break down overly dualistic conceptualisation of patients' problems
- Excellent opportunity to train non-psychiatric trainees in psychiatric and psychological aspects of their speciality
- Improves assessment as it is not so dependent on the physician's detection of psychiatric problems

Disadvantages

- Complicated to set up, as times need to be coordinated and sufficient clinic rooms identified
- It may prove to be a relatively expensive way to run services and an inefficient use of specialist time
- Integrated services challenge the traditional ways of working of both parties and may in the short term disrupt effective working practices

Out-patient services – conclusions

Four main ways of working with psychiatric out-patients in general hospitals have been presented. All have advantages and disadvantages. On the basis of his experience working in the Seattle pain clinic, Sullivan (1993) has strongly advocated the integrated clinic as the best model for fostering cooperation between clinicians and for maximising patient acceptance of a psychiatric or psychological contribution to their management. However, there is no doubt that this form of joint working is the most difficult to organise.

Overall conclusions

What style of working should we pursue?

We would suggest that rather than choosing a single model, a combination of working styles is employed. There needs to be an emergency consultation service for acutely disturbed or suicidal patients, including patients admitted following deliberate self-harm. In addition, a specialist liaison psychiatry/psychology out-patient clinic will almost certainly be necessary for complex cases to allow sufficient time to conduct detailed assessment interviews and to provide ongoing treatment. However, these ways of working do not challenge the traditional and unhelpful division between medicine/surgery and psychiatry/psychology. Also, both depend on the non-psychiatrist's ability to select patients for referral.

We suggest therefore that, in addition to the above, efforts be made to establish more integrated working. The simplest form is regular liaison between the psychiatrist and specific units. More demanding would be the setting up of a single joint medical/psychiatric out-patient clinic to which the general practitioner could refer complex cases. Finally, for a small number of patients the argument is over-whelming for jointly managed beds staffed by nurses who can manage combined medical and psychiatric problems; in practice, this is difficult. It will be interesting to see whether any such beds are funded in the UK National Health Service.

Who pays?

In a cash-strapped National Health Service, each speciality can readily develop a siege mentality. Those who try to set up joint ventures may encounter difficulty in obtaining agreement about whether medical or psychiatric budgets will meet the cost. There is a case for arguing that the medical service budget should cover the provision of a comprehensive service for its patients. There is also a case for arguing that the psychiatric budget should be set on the understanding that physical illness must not be a barrier to receiving good mental health care. There is no case for failing to identify the budget for this group of patients, who are at double jeopardy.

References

BARSKY, A. J. (1983) Overview: hypochondriasis, bodily complaints, and somatic styles. *American Journal of Psychiatry*, **140**, 273–283.

BASLER, H. D., JAKLE, C. & KRONER-HERWIG, B. (1997) Incorporation of cognitive–behavioural treatment into the medical care of chronic low back patients: a controlled randomised study in German pain treatment centres. *Patient Education and Counselling*, **31**, 113–124.

DOLINAR, L. J. (1993) A historical review of outpatient consultation–liaison psychiatry. *General Hospital Psychiatry*, **15**, 363–368.

FINK, P. (1992) The use of hospitalisations by persistent somatising patients. *Psychological Medicine*, **22**, 173–180.

HAMILTON, J., CAMPOS, R. & CREED, F. (1996) Anxiety, depression and the management of medically unexplained symptoms in medical clinics. *Journal of the Royal College of Physicians, London*, **30**, 18–20.

HARSCH, H. H., KORAN, L. M. & YOUNG, L. D. (1991) A profile of academic medical–psychiatric units. *General Hospital Psychiatry*, **13**, 291–295.

HAWTON, K. E. (1996) Self-poisoning and the general hospital. *Quarterly Journal of Medicine*, **89**, 879–880.

HERTZOG, T. (1991) Inpatient treatment of patients with severe neurotic and psychosomatic disorders: a German perspective. *British Journal of Psychotherapy*, **8**, 189–198.

HOUSE, A. (1995) Editorial. Psychiatric disorders, inappropriate health service utilisation and the role of consultation–liaison psychiatry. *Journal of Psychosomatic Research*, **39**, 799–802.

HUYSE, F. J., STRAIN, J. J. & HAMMER, J. S. (1990) Interventions in consultation/liaison psychiatry. Part II: Concordance. *General Hospital Psychiatry*, **12**, 221–231.

KATHOL, R. G., HARSCH, H. H., HALL, R. C., *et al* (1992) Categorization of types of medical/psychiatry units based on level of acuity. *Psychosomatics*, **33**, 376–386.

KIRMAYER, L. J. (1988) Mind and body as metaphors: hidden values in biomedicine. In *Biomedicine Examined* (eds M. Lock & D. Gordon), pp. 57–92. Dordrecht: Kluwer.

LIN, E. H., KATON, W. J., VON KORFF, M., *et al* (1991) Frustrating patients: physician and patient perspectives among distressed high utilisers of medical services. *Journal of General Internal Medicine*, **6**, 241–246.

MAYOU, R. A., ANDERSON, H., FEINMANN, C., *et al* (1990) The present state of consultation and liaison psychiatry. *Psychiatric Bulletin*, **14**, 321–325.

—— & SHARPE, M. (1995) Psychiatric illness associated with physical disease. *Baillière's Clinical Psychiatry*, **1**, 201–224.

——, BASS, C. & SHARPE, M. (1995) *Treatment of Functional Somatic Symptoms*. Oxford: Oxford University Press.

PERSSON, J. & MAGNUSSON, P. H. (1987) Prevalence of excessive or problem drinkers among patients attending somatic outpatient clinics: a study of alcohol related medical care. *British Medical Journal*, **295**, 467–472.

PETERS, A. A., VAN DORST, E., JELLIS, B., *et al* (1991) A randomised clinical trial to compare two different approaches in women with chronic pelvic pain. *Obstetrics and Gynaecology*, **77**, 740–744.

SCHWEITZER, R., ROBERTSON, D. L., KELLY, B., *et al* (1994) Illness behaviour of patients with chronic fatigue syndrome. *Journal of Psychosomatic Research*, **38**, 41–49.

SHARPE, M., MAYOU, R. A., SEAGROTT, V., *et al* (1994) Why do doctors find some patients difficult to help? *Quarterly Journal of Medicine*, **87**, 187–193.

SULLIVAN, M. D. (1993) Psychosomatic clinic or pain clinic – which is more viable? *General Hospital Psychiatry*, **15**, 375–380.

WILLIAMS, A., NICHOLAS, M. K., RICHARDSON, P. H., *et al* (1993) Evaluation of a cognitive behavioural programme for rehabilitating patients with chronic pain. *British Journal of General Practice*, **43**, 513–518.

Index

216 *Index*